T0192125

Rural Nursing
The Australian context

The Australian rural environment is unique, diverse and challenging for nurses who are the most significant providers of health care in this context. *Rural Nursing: The Australian context* provides readers with an understanding of the knowledge and skills required to practise in rural locations and communities.

In recognition of the need for rural nurses to be versatile and knowledgeable in every aspect of health care, this book includes chapters on pregnancy, parenting, childhood, adolescence, adulthood, ageing and mental health. It examines rurality, population and health demographics, and the different practice opportunities available in rural settings. The authors outline the importance of having well-established professional networks and encourage readers to develop practice skills in response to a particular community. Chapters feature vignettes, reflective questions and lists of websites for further reading.

Written by a team of academics and practising rural nurses, *Rural Nursing* will equip nursing students with the confidence to provide high-quality health care in a range of practice settings.

Karen Francis is Professor in the School of Nursing, Midwifery and Indigenous Health at Charles Sturt University, Wagga Wagga.

Ysanne Chapman is an independent scholar and has adjunct professor status with James Cook University, Charles Sturt University, Monash University and Adelaide University.

Carmel Davies is Lecturer in the School of Nursing, Midwifery and Indigenous Health at Charles Sturt University, Wagga Wagga.

Rural Nursing
The Australian
context

Edited by

Karen Francis   *Ysanne Chapman*   *Carmel Davies*

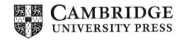

CAMBRIDGE
UNIVERSITY PRESS

University Printing House, Cambridge CB2 8BS, United Kingdom

One Liberty Plaza, 20th Floor, New York, NY 10006, USA

477 Williamstown Road, Port Melbourne, VIC 3207, Australia

314-321, 3rd Floor, Plot 3, Splendor Forum, Jasola District Centre, New Delhi - 110025, India

79 Anson Road, #06-04/06, Singapore 079906

Cambridge University Press is part of the University of Cambridge.

It furthers the University's mission by disseminating knowledge in the pursuit of education, learning and research at the highest international levels of excellence.

www.cambridge.org
Information on this title: www.cambridge.org/9781107626829

First published 2014

Cover designed by Kerry Cooke
Typeset by Aptara Corp.

A catalogue record for this publication is available from the British Library

A Cataloguing-in-Publication entry is available from the catalogue of the National Library of Australia at www.nla.gov.au

ISBN 978-1-107-62682-9 Paperback

....

Every effort has been made in preparing this book to provide accurate and up-to-date information which is in accord with accepted standards and practice at the time of publication. Although case histories are drawn from actual cases, every effort has been made to disguise the identities of the individuals involved. Nevertheless, the authors, editors and publishers can make no warranties that the information contained herein is totally free from error, not least because clinical standards are constantly changing through research and regulation. The authors, editors and publishers therefore disclaim all liability for direct or consequential damages resulting from the use of material contained in this book. Readers are strongly advised to pay careful attention to information provided by the manufacturer of any drugs or equipment that they plan to use.

Contents

11 Conclusion: sustaining the health of rural populations 176

Karen Francis, Ysanne Chapman, Faye McMillan and Jane Havelka

Contributors

Judith Anderson is Senior Lecturer and Postgraduate Program Leader in the School of Nursing, Midwifery & Indigenous Health at Charles Sturt University.

Melanie Birks is Professor of Nursing, Teaching and Learning in the School of Nursing, Midwifery & Nutrition at James Cook University, Townsville campus. Her academic career has spanned most of the past two decades.

Angela Bradley is Head of School at Navitas, Health Skills Australia. She has 20 years' experience in academia and regulatory positions and 10 in clinical practice focused predominantly on child health. She is currently undertaking her PhD.

Ann-Marie Brown is Lecturer in Nursing and also Clinical Coordinator in the School of Nursing, Midwifery & Indigenous Health at Charles Sturt University.

Ysanne Chapman is Adjunct Professor at James Cook University, Charles Sturt University, Monash University and the University of Adelaide. She has had a long and varied career in nursing academe and works from home in Victoria as an independent scholar.

Carmel Davies is Lecturer in the School of Nursing, Midwifery & Indigenous Health at Charles Sturt University. She has worked in the tertiary sector for many years, teaching and researching in nursing and aged care in rural areas.

Jenny Davis is a Monash University PhD candidate currently working as Project Manager on a large Department of Social Services grant examining innovation models that improve older person service access and health outcomes. She is a nurse and midwife with many years' experience in the Australian healthcare sector as clinician, manager, educator and researcher.

Sally Drummond is a credentialled mental health nurse and lecturer in the School of Nursing, Midwifery & Indigenous Health at Charles Sturt University. She has worked in the tertiary education and mental health sectors for many years.

Mary FitzGerald is Professor of Nursing in the School of Nursing, Midwifery & Indigenous Health at Charles Sturt University. She has experience as both a clinician and a nursing academic. Her early research centred around the experience of chronic illness in rural Australia.

Karen Francis is Professor and Head of the School of Nursing, Midwifery & Indigenous Health at Charles Sturt University. She has been Chair of the Australian College of Nursing, Rural Nursing and Midwifery Faculty, and President, Australian Rural Nurses and Midwives (ARNM) and President, Association of Australian Rural Nurses (AARN).

Peta Lea Gale is Lecturer at the Australian Catholic University. Prior to this she worked in paediatric acute care, specialising in cardiac renal nursing.

Jane Havelka is a Wiradjuri woman from Narromine Wongabon currently residing in Wagga Wagga, New South Wales. She is Clinical Coordinator/Lecturer for the Djirruwang (Mental Health) Program in the School of Nursing, Midwifery & Indigenous Health at Charles Sturt University. Jane is a Director on the Board of Indigenous Allied Health Australia (IAHA).

Desley Hegney is Professor of Nursing in the School of Nursing and Midwifery at Curtin University. She is the inaugural President of the Western Australian Honor Society of Nursing (affiliated with Sigma Theta Tau International [STTI]).

Ainsley James is Clinical Coordinator at Federation University Gippsland (formerly Monash University Gippsland), where she teaches undergraduate nursing and midwifery. She has 13 years' clinical experience in rural Victoria and nine years in academia.

Margaret McLeod is Associate Head of the School of Nursing, Midwifery & Indigenous Health at Charles Sturt University, where she is responsible for school activities at Wagga Wagga and Albury campuses.

Faye McMillan is a Wiradjuri woman from Trangie, Central Western New South Wales. She is the Director of the Djirruwang Program in the School of Nursing, Midwifery & Indigenous Health at Charles Sturt University, Wagga Wagga campus. Faye is the Chairperson of Indigenous Allied Health Australia (IAHA).

Maureen Miles is a midwife, nurse, and maternal and child health nurse. She lectures in midwifery and coordinates the midwifery program in the School of Nursing and Midwifery at Federation University Australia.

Jane Mills is Associate Professor and Director of the Centre for Nursing and Midwifery Research and Associate Dean (Research) in the Faculty of Medicine, Health and Molecular Sciences at James Cook University.

John Rosenberg is a researcher with the Supportive and Palliative Care Team at Queensland University of Technology and Adjunct Associate Professor in the School of Nursing, Midwifery & Indigenous Health at Charles Sturt University. He is a registered nurse with a clinical background in community-based palliative care.

Moira Williamson is Associate Professor and Head of Midwifery Programs at Central Queensland University. She has extensive experience as a midwife and midwifery manager.

Acknowledgements

I would like to acknowledge the contribution of each of the authors who have contributed and the people from whom they have drawn inspiration. My thanks to my personal assistant, Ms Holly Gray, who has had the dubious pleasure of living through the creation of this text. Her ability to solve my never ending computer problems, access information and resources, and make sense of my cryptic requests never ceases to amaze me. Finally, I acknowledge the man behind the scenes, my husband who is always there and listens, I think, whenever I complain about taking on too much.

Karen Francis

I wish to thank all the contributors to this first edition. It is exciting to be part of a new text on rural nursing. In particular I would like to say thank you to my two colleagues, Karen and Carmel. I have had the pleasure of writing with Karen on numerous occasions; one more text is another success in a long line of publications. Over the years I have learned much from Carmel's expertise with words and this publication has been just as inspiring.

Ysanne Chapman

Numerous people have contributed to this book; too many to acknowledge each one individually. But I would like to particularly thank each contributor for their hard work and excellent contributions. I should also mention the rewarding experience gained through working with my fellow editors on this project.

Carmel Davies

1 The context

Karen Francis and Ysanne Chapman

Learning objectives

On completion of this chapter, the reader will be able to:

- describe an overview of the history and culture of the Australian population

- discuss the statistics of the Australian population

- describe the current health priorities for Australia

- provide an overview of how health care is provided in Australia and how the various governments impact on health policy development

- source how education of healthcare workers is provided in Australia.

Key words

Australia, health policy, population, healthcare worker, education provider

Chapter overview

This chapter provides background to the text. The Australian population, legislative frameworks and policies, health challenges and health priorities are described. A profile of the health workforce in Australia is included.

Background

Australia is an ancient island continent covering 7 682 300 square kilometres (Australian Government, 2013b) and is the world's sixth largest country (Tourism Australia, 2013a). The traditional peoples of this land arrived approximately 50 000 years ago from South-East Asia during the last Ice Age (Tourism Australia, 2013b). These peoples dispersed across the land, adapting their ways of life to accommodate the bounty offered and developing unique languages and cultures (Australian Bureau of Statistics [ABS], 2013a). The Indigenous peoples established tribal lands and trade partners with neighbouring groups. Kinship ties were formalised as members of the neighbouring groups established relationships that bound tribes and clans together (Indigenous Australia, 2013).

Archaeological evidence suggests that the northern borders of Australia were regularly visited by traders from South-East Asia who contributed to the diversity of the Indigenous populations (ABS, 2013a). European sailors also visited Australia prior to Captain James Cook claiming Australia for England in 1778. Willem Janszoon travelled from Indonesia to Cape York Peninsula in 1606, and Dirk Hartog, another Dutch explorer, came ashore on the west coast of Australia in 1615 and probably interacted with local peoples. Hartog's discovery of the 'Great Southern Land' led to its inclusion in world maps of the time and facilitated increased expeditions by other European sailors (Australian history, 2013). Abel Tasman, another Dutch sailor, is acknowledged for his 'discovery' of Tasmania, which he named Van Diemens Land. La Perouse, a French explorer, was engaged by the French Admiralty to seek out and claim new lands and trade partners for France (Morrisey, 1924). He arrived in Botany Bay two days after Captain James Cook, who was commissioned by the British Admiralty and the Royal Society to take an expedition to Tahiti to record the transit of Venus. In addition, Cook was instructed to travel to New Zealand and then to the 'Great Southern Land' to chart these land masses for future exploration. He was also charged with identifying the potential for trade or extracting resources of interest such as timber and flax for ships' sails and with laying claim for the Crown of new worlds (Museum of New Zealand Te Papa Tongarewa, 2013).

Following his success, the white colonisation of Australia occurred in 1788 with the arrival of the First Fleet (Australian Government, 2013c). History records that initial relationships between the traditional owners of Australia and the colonisers were affable, with trade occurring; however, hostility grew as land was usurped by the colonisers (Australian Government, 2013c). Conflict between the Indigenous peoples of Australia and the white colonisers featured in the subsequent history of Australia.

Australia is, by history and intentional colonial claim, a multicultural nation, bringing together people from Europe, Melanesia and within itself. How this diversity manifested itself and how our culture was realised is the substance of the following section.

Culture

Australian culture is as broad and varied as the country's landscape. Australia is multicultural and multiracial, and this is reflected in its food, lifestyle and cultural practices and experience. Indigenous people, as the traditional custodians of the lands, have an important heritage that plays a defining role in the Australian cultural landscape (Australian Government, 2013d).

This diversity of influences has resulted in a cultural environment that is described by Tourism Australia as lively, energised, innovative and outward looking (2013a). The folklore of the nation has evolved from the Indigenous influence of telling stories. Traditionally, Indigenous Australians shared their heritage and explained understandings of their world through dreamtime and creation stories, oral histories spoken of between families and groups, and through art and dance. Even the life stories of the earliest colonists – many of whom were of Irish descent, the military and convicts transported by the British Government in the 18th and 19th centuries for crimes against the Crown – have been shared and passed on through the generations. These experiences and those of infamous characters who have called Australia home (including Ned Kelly, Captain Lightfoot and explorers who journeyed into the uncharted reaches of the land to discover it), as well as the men and women who have given their lives in times of war and the immigrants who have come to Australia seeking a better life, have all contributed to the rich tapestry of culture that is uniquely Australian (Tourism Australia, 2013a).

Culture in health and illness influences the perception and meanings of health, illness and healing practices and how healthcare information and treatments are received. Understanding and recognising the centrality of culture for Aboriginal and Torres Strait Islander people, which also extends to many other cultures within the Australian landscape, are critical to health practitioners being culturally responsive to the environments in which service delivery occurs. Indigenous Allied Health Australia (IAHA) views cultural responsiveness as an extension of patient-centred care that pays particular attention to social and cultural factors in managing therapeutic encounters with patients from different cultural and social backgrounds (IAHA, 2013). IAHA (2013) also asserts that cultural responsiveness is a cyclical and ongoing process requiring health professionals to continuously self-reflect and proactively respond to the person, family or community with whom they interact. What is healthy in one culture may not be so in another, and vice versa (Harvey & Park, 2011).

There are several initiatives focused on Australian culture that guide health care, and some government departments and professional organisations that provide this direction are:

- Immigration Health Advisory Group (IHAG)
- National Strategic Framework for Aboriginal and Torres Strait Islander Health 2003–2013
- National Health and Hospitals Reform Commission (NHHRC)
- The National Advisory Group on Aboriginal and Torres Strait Islander Health Information and Data (NAGATSIHID)
- Congress of Aboriginal and Torres Strait Islander Nurses (CATSIN)
- Australian Indigenous Doctors' Association (AIDA)
- National Congress of Australia's First Peoples
- Indigenous Allied Health Australia (IAHA)
- Close the Gap campaign
- Council of Australian Governments (COAG) Closing the Gap in Indigenous Disadvantage (Harvey & Park, 2011).

Culture is one of the determinants of health. As we will see later in the chapter, the population of Australia largely hugs the coastline, and those living in rural areas do not share the same access and equity to health services. Thus, being from a different culture to the mainstream and living in rural or remote locations can impact negatively on access to health services. As we progress through the text, we will spend some time discussing the impact of these and other issues on the health of rural dwellers.

Population

The population of Australia was 23 044 766 as at 5 June 2013 (ABS, 2013f). The ABS reported that the Australian population grew by 1.7% during the year 2012. This growth was a result of a natural increase of 40%. A growth of 60% could be attributed to overseas migration (ABS, 2013b). Data from 2011 indicate that there are slightly more female (11.2 million) than male (11.1 million) Australians. The ratio of males to females, however, is greater outside the capital cities, with the greatest difference occurring in the outback of Western Australia, Queensland and the Northern Territory (see Figure 1.1) (ABS, 2013c).

The majority of the population resides on the coastal fringes in the major capitals of each state or territory. Sydney, New South Wales, and Melbourne, Victoria, are the largest cities in the most populous states in Australia (Tourism

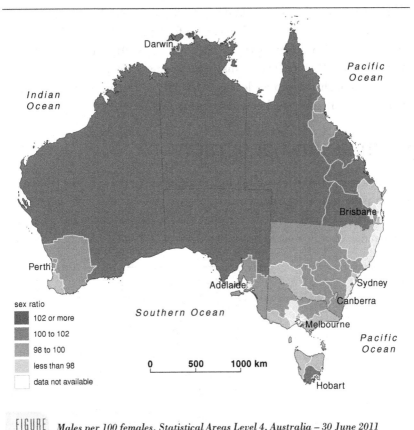

FIGURE 1.1 *Males per 100 females, Statistical Areas Level 4, Australia – 30 June 2011 (ABS, 2013c).*

Australia, 2013a). Recent data indicate that the population has grown in Western Australia, which is probably in part related to the expansion of the mining industry (ABS, 2013g).

Morbidity and mortality data indicate that the major causes of death for Australians are circulatory diseases and cancers (AIHW, 2013a). The ABS reported that, by the 1970s, the incidence of death from circulatory system diseases was declining, offering improved lifestyles as a rationale for this trend. The ABS asserted that the incidence of cancer-related deaths is rising, and that this trend is related to increased longevity of the population. Male deaths from cancers are higher than for females, with males dying from trachea, bronchus and lung cancers that have been linked to tobacco smoking (ABS, 2013d).

Infant mortality rates are 4.55 deaths/1000 live births, with male infant rates (4.87/1000 live births) slightly higher than for female infants (4.21/1000 live births) (Australian infant mortality rate, 2013). In 2010, Indigenous infant mortality rates (7/1000 live births) were greater than for non-Indigenous infants, although the gap is closing (ABS, 2013e; Department of Families, Housing, Community Services & Indigenous Affairs, 2013).

Climate and geography

Australia is situated between the Indian and Pacific Oceans. The land mass is approximately 4000 kilometres from east to west and 3200 kilometres from north to south, with a coastline 36 735 kilometres long. Climatic zones range from tropical rainforests, deserts (20% of the land continent),

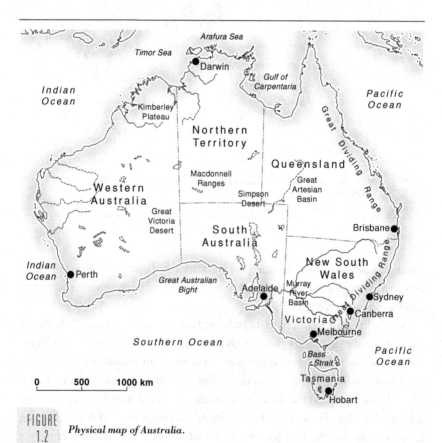

FIGURE
1.2   *Physical map of Australia.*

cool temperature forests and snow-covered mountains (Australian Government, 2013b). Figure 1.2 provides details of the physical features of the Australian landscape.

Australia's climate is varied depending on geographic location (latitude). The northern regions have a tropical climate, while the southern states have a more temperate climate. As the majority of the continent is arid (apart from the coastal fringes and Tasmania), Australia is the world's second driest continent. Summer temperatures are high and winters mild and warm in the north (ABS, 2013d). Rainfall varies, with the highest average rainfall on the east coast of Queensland between Cairns and Cardwell. Figure 1.3 details average rainfall for Australia 1961–1990. The least rainfall during this period was in the arid centre.

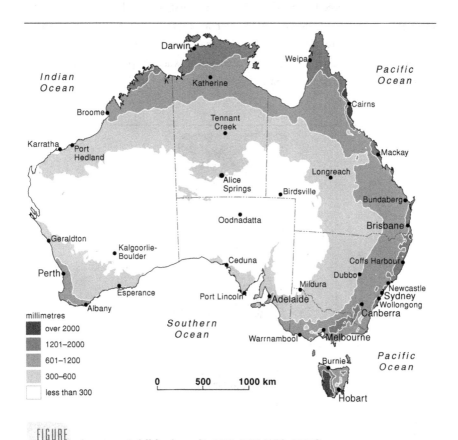

FIGURE 1.3 *Average rainfall for Australia 1961–1990 (ABS, 2013d).*

The government of Australia

Australia, as a former British colony, has remained a member of the Commonwealth of Nations (formally known as the British Commonwealth of Nations). As such, Australia's Government is a constitutional monarchy. Australia recognises Queen Elizabeth II as the Head of State. The Head of State has the power to appoint a Governor-General who acts on her behalf. The powers of government are defined by a constitution that came into force on 1 January 1901; a date referred to as the 'Birth of the Nation'. On this date, six colonies – namely Western Australia, South Australia, Tasmania, Victoria, New South Wales and Queensland – agreed to form a federated nation. A central government was formed that has the power to pass laws that pertain to the whole of the country, as decreed in Section 51 of the Constitution. The state/territory governments have legislative power over all matters occurring within their jurisdictions and are able to establish local governments to manage local matters such as housing, water, roads, sewage and waste disposal (see Figure 1.4) (Australian Government, 2013a).

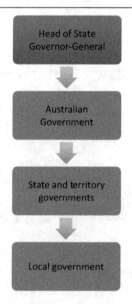

FIGURE 1.4 *Government structure in Australia (Australian Government, 2013a).*

Federal/Australian Government

The Australian Government is elected on a three-year cycle and is responsible for:

- taxation
- defence
- foreign affairs
- postal and telecommunications services
- state and territory governments (Australian Government, 2013a).

State and territory governments

The state and territory governments have responsibility for matters that are restricted to their boundaries, such as:

- police
- hospitals
- education
- public transport (Australian Government, 2013a).

Local government

The final level in the Australian system of government is local government. Local governments are established by state and territory governments and have responsibility for a range of community services (Australian Government, 2013a).

Global and national health policy

Australia, like most nations, views access to health care as a basic human right (Podger & Hagan, 1999). Providing for the health and safety of the nation has been a feature of Australian governments since white colonisation. All levels of government have a role in supporting health care in Australia. The Australian Government directly funds medicine (general practice and specialists) and aged care and has recently taken on responsibility for the regulation of health professionals (Commonwealth Fund, 2013; Podger & Hagan, 1999). State governments are responsible for the delivery of public health services (hospital and community) and the regulation of private hospitals. Local governments manage public health services such as some child and maternal health services, and parenting services. All Australians have access to health care through Medicare, a national health insurance scheme funded through taxation revenue by the Australian Government. The Medical Benefits Scheme, also funded by the Australian Government, subsidises medications that are listed on a formulary (Francis, Chapman, Hoare & Birks, 2013).

In response to spiralling healthcare costs and recognition that the traditional model of health care was intervention focused, the Australian Government revised the national health priorities, identifying primary care and preventative health care as the way forward (AIHW, 2013a). The World Health Organization has influenced health policy and service delivery in Australia, and this has led to the rethinking and shaping of the national health priorities. The national health priorities for Australia in 2013 were:

- Cancer control
  - The most common causes of cancer deaths in 2010 were lung cancer (8099 deaths), bowel cancer (3982 deaths), prostate cancer (3235 deaths), breast cancer (2864 deaths) and pancreatic cancer (2434 deaths). Survival rates for cancer have significantly improved over time, and 66% of people with cancer survived in 2010 compared with 47% in 1987 (AIHW, 2013a).
- Cardiovascular health
  - The main types of cardiovascular disease (CVD) in Australia are coronary heart disease, stroke, heart failure and cardiomyopathy, acute rheumatic fever and rheumatic heart disease, peripheral vascular disease and congenital heart disease. Approximately 17% of the Australian population have CVD and, although the disease is common for men, it is rapidly becoming a disease found in women of all ages. Rheumatic heart disease is more common in the Indigenous population (AIHW, 2013a).
- Injury prevention and control
  - Injury contributes significantly to the burden of disease, and in 2010 it was assessed to be 6.5% of the total burden of disease in Australia. Approximately 400 000 people undergo an injury yearly, severe enough to be hospitalised. Older females have higher rates of injury as a result of falls. The rates of all injury, however, have been constant since 2000 (AIHW, 2013a).
- Mental health
  - Mental ill-health accounts for 24% of total years lost because of disability in Australia. Mental ill-health is the fastest growing illness factor in

Australia. The *2007 National Survey of Mental Health and Wellbeing* (ABS as cited in AIHW, 2013a) found that 3.2 million Australians had a mental illness in the 12 months prior to the survey. This statistic equates to 20% of the population aged between 16 and 85 years (AIHW, 2013a).

- Diabetes mellitus
  - Approximately 4% of all Australians suffer from diabetes mellitus. This figure represents 898 000 people – a rise from 1.5% in 1989. Data estimate that 87 100 suffer from type 1 diabetes and 787 500 suffer from type 2. Diabetes is more common in the Indigenous population than in the non-Indigenous population, and its prevalence increases with age (AIHW, 2013a).
- Asthma
  - In 2003, 61% of the burden of disease attributed to asthma was said to be in children aged 0–14 years. The prevalence of asthma in younger children has led to the rise of Asthma Friendly Schools in Australia (AIHW, 2013a).
- Arthritis and musculoskeletal conditions
  - Musculoskeletal conditions are the most common chronic conditions affecting almost one-third of the population. Musculoskeletal conditions are defined as conditions of the bones, muscles and their attachments, such as joints. A total of 1.6 million Australians suffer from osteoarthritis, whereas 428 000 are affected by rheumatoid arthritis. In addition, 1.9 million report some form of back problem (AIHW, 2013a).
- Obesity
  - In Australia, three in five adults are overweight. Being overweight is a major risk factor for CVD, type 2 diabetes, some musculoskeletal conditions and some cancers. More people living in rural and remote areas are overweight than people in major cities. The main cause of obesity is the imbalance between energy in and energy out. Energy requirements fluctuate with age and physical expenditure. Attention to food and drink consumption is a priority for anyone who wants to maintain a healthy weight regime. Large body mass was responsible for 7.2% of total deaths in Australia in 2003; this figure equates to 9500 people (AIHW, 2013a).
- Dementia
  - Dementia is a general term that describes a number of different illnesses that lead to a decline in mental or cognitive function. The most well known of the dementias is Alzheimer's disease. Dementia is an illness that is rapidly increasing in prevalence, mostly because of the ageing

of the population. In fact, the main risk factor for dementia is age. In Australia, the 2006 estimated prevalence of dementia was 1% of those aged 60–65 years, 6% of those aged 75–79 years and 45% of those aged 95 years or more (Alzheimer's Australia, 2005).

These priorities demand that effective preventative health care is seen as the panacea of policy. This focus is true for world health issues. There has been little change in global health issues since 2001 – the main areas needing to be addressed are the elimination of infectious diseases (malaria and tuberculosis being the main protagonists), the control of HIV, the improvement of world nutrition and immunisation and vaccination programs, and the lowering of maternal and perinatal mortality rates (Olila, 2005).

No matter what health priorities are identified, their management and the care of people whose health is compromised lie in the remit of healthcare workers.

Health workforce

The Australian health workforce is diverse, consisting of regulated and unregulated (e.g. nurse assistants, residential care workers, health workers) healthcare workers. Regulated health professionals include nurses, midwives, doctors, and a range of allied and complementary health providers. This group of health professionals has grown exponentially since 2001 (AIHW, 2013b), and that development in itself has increased the cost of the provision of health care. The distribution of this group of health professionals is not evenly dispersed across the nation, with the largest concentration of providers being located in the capital cities and highly populated regions. The exception is nursing, which is relatively evenly distributed across all geographic classifications (Health Workforce Australia [HWA], 2012a), although there are current workforce shortages in this group. Predictions suggest that shortages will worsen if methods to promote recruitment and retention of nurses are not implemented. HWA is advocating for the advancement of nursing practice as an initiative to improve access to health care and as a recruitment and retention strategy (2012b). HWA is a statutory authority established by the Australian Government to coordinate a national approach to workforce reform. This agency:

> … has been working in collaboration with governments and non-government organisations across health and higher education sectors to address critical priorities in the planning, training and reform of Australia's health workforce (HWA, 2013, para 2).

Health workforce education

The focus by the Australian Government on the health workforce is in response to recognised shortages and misdistribution of some health professional groups (doctors and allied health). Increasing the numbers of students in targeted health programs such as nursing has been one strategy adopted to address the predicted shortages. The Australian Health Practitioner Regulation Agency (AHPRA) works with 14 health professional regulatory boards to regulate and accredit members. The 14 boards are:

- Aboriginal and Torres Strait Islander Health Practice Board of Australia
- Chinese Medicine Board of Australia
- Chiropractic Board of Australia
- Dental Board of Australia
- Medical Board of Australia
- Medical Radiation Practice Board of Australia
- Nursing and Midwifery Board of Australia
- Occupational Therapy Board of Australia
- Optometry Board of Australia
- Osteopathy Board of Australia
- Pharmacy Board of Australia
- Physiotherapy Board of Australia
- Podiatry Board of Australia
- Psychology Board of Australia (AHPRA, 2013).

Nursing education

Educational programs leading to the licensure in any of the professions covered by these boards are accredited and monitored by AHPRA. In Australia, there are two levels of regulated nurses: registered and enrolled nurses. The Australian Nursing and Midwifery Accreditation Council (ANMAC) oversees the management of accreditation through a process of stringent peer review against the professionally agreed framework and competencies of the two levels of licensure. Tertiary education providers (usually universities) deliver accredited programs of study leading to registered nurse licensure (ANMAC, 2010). Pre-service programs leading to registration as a registered nurse include three- to four-year bachelor level degrees and postgraduate 'entry to practice' master's degrees. Enrolled nurses undertake diploma level studies offered by vocational education sector providers (TAFE).

Education providers are concentrated in the capital cities, although there are regional universities located in some regional and rural environments. Many of these providers have tailored their programs to include information on regional and rural issues and clinical practice exposure in regional and rural settings to ensure that graduates are equipped for practice in these locales (ANMAC, 2010). In recent years the establishment of clinical schools, particularly in rural locations by primarily medical faculties, has supported clinical rotations of students to sites that were not utilised in the past. Access to accommodation and appropriate supervision for some students in rural and regional areas are issues that have been resolved with the establishment of clinical schools. However, these solutions are not translated to other health professionals, and nurses and allied healthcare workers often incur significant extra costs for undertaking rural and remote clinical placements in their respective degree programs.

VIGNETTE

Sally is a Year 12 student who lives on the edge of a rural town in New South Wales, 550 kilometres south west of Sydney. She dreams of becoming a nurse and securing a job as a registered nurse in a general practice setting. She lives with her parents, her three older brothers and two younger sisters on a sheep station. Her father and brothers work the sheep station while her sisters are in Year 10 and Year 9 at the high school Sally attends. Sally is the only person in her immediate family who has the ability or desire to go to university. Her younger sister has secured a hairdressing apprenticeship after Year 10, and her youngest sister wants to work in a shop. The closest university offering nursing as a three-year degree or a four-year double degree with midwifery is located 480 kilometres from home. Sally has never left home before and, as the eldest daughter, her mother has relied on her to help in the home and with the meals at shearing time. Sally also suffers from chronic asthma, which is controlled by preventer medication. Her asthma worsens on exertion and at season change.

Questions
1 What motivators does Sally have to fulfil her life's dream?
2 What challenges would she face leaving home?
3 What challenges will the family face if Sally leaves home?
4 How might Sally ensure her job desires are realised?
5 What sorts of decisions do Sally and her parents have to make to send Sally to university?
6 As a registered nurse, what ideas might you give Sally to manage her asthma while she is at university?

Summary

In this first chapter, we have set the scene of living in rural Australia. We have described how rural Australia was settled, the culture of living and working in a rural town, the healthcare system of Australia and the national health priorities. Lastly, we provide a scenario of Sally, a rural Australian girl who wants to become a nurse, and we ask you to focus on the various family issues and challenges Sally might face if she is successful in pursuing her choice of study.

In this chapter, we have covered:

- the Australian population
- health policy
- health challenges and national health priorities
- health workforce.

Reflective questions

1 Discuss the uniqueness of the Australian landscape and the impact on settlement.
2 Consider the Australian population. Discuss the impact of cultural heritage on contemporary Australia.
3 Review the Australian Government structure and identify the responsibilities of each level of government.
4 List the national health priorities and discuss the implications for health services.
5 Consider the Australian health workforce: what contribution do nurses and midwives make?

References

Alzheimer's Australia. (2005). Annual Report 2004/2005. Scullin ACT: Alzheimer's Australia. Retrieved May 28, 2013, from http://www.fightdementia.org.au/research-publications/alzheimers-australia-annual-reports.aspx

Australian Bureau of Statistics. (2013a). *Unity and diversity: The history and culture of Aboriginal Australia*. Canberra: Australian Government. Retrieved May 3, 2013, from http://www.abs.gov.au/Ausstats/abs@.nsf/0/75258e92a5903e75ca2569de0025c188?OpenDocument

——. (2013b). 310.0 – *Australian demographic statistics, Sept 2012*. Canberra: Australian Government. Retrieved May 6, 2013, from http://www.abs.gov.au/ausstats/abs@.nsf/mf/3101.0

——. (2013c). 3235.0 – *Population by age and sex, regions of Australia, 2011*. Canberra: Australian Government. Retrieved May 6, 2013, from http://www.abs.gov.au/ausstats/abs@.nsf/Products/3235.0~2011~Main+Features~Main+Features?OpenDocument

——. (2013d). 4102.0 – *Australian social trends, 2011*. Canberra: Australian Government. Retrieved May 6, 2013, from http://www.abs.gov.au/ausstats/abs@.nsf/2f762f95845417aeca25706c00834efa/45feea54e2403635ca2570ec000c46e1!OpenDocument

——. (2013e). 4704.0 – *The health and welfare of Australia's Aboriginal and Torres Strait Islander peoples, Oct 2010.* Canberra: Australian Government. Retrieved May 6, 2013, from http://www.abs.gov.au/ausstats/abs@.nsf/Lookup/4704.0

——. (2013f). *Population clock.* Canberra: Australian Government. Retrieved June 5, 2013, from http://www.abs.gov.au/ausstats/abs%40.nsf/94713ad445ff1425ca256 82000192af2/1647509ef7e25faaca2568a900154b63?OpenDocument

——. (2013g). *Towns of the mining boom.* Canberra: Australian Government. Retrieved May 6, 2013, from http://www.abs.gov.au/AUSSTATS/abs@.nsf/ Lookup/4102.0Main+Features10April+2013

Australian Government. (2013a). *Australia's federation.* Canberra: Australian Government. Retrieved May 7, 2013, from http://australia.gov.au/about-australia/our-government/australias-federation

——. (2013b). *The Australian continent.* Canberra: Australian Government. Retrieved May 7, 2013, from http://australia.gov.au/about-australia/our-country/the-australian-continent

——. (2013c). *European discovery and the colonisation of Australia.* Canberra: Australian Government. Retrieved May 6, 2013, from http://australia.gov.au/ about-australia/australian-story/european-discovery-and-colonisation

——. (2013d). *Our country.* Canberra: Australian Government. Retrieved May 6, 2013, from http://australia.gov.au/about-australia/our-country

Australian Health Practitioner Regulation Agency (AHPRA). (2013). About AHPRA. Canberra: AHPRA. Retrieved May 15, 2013, from http://www.ahpra. gov.au/About-AHPRA.aspx

Australian history: Dirk Hartog. (2013). Canberra. Retrieved May 6, 2013, from http://www.australianhistory.org/dirk-hartog

Australian infant mortality rate. (2013). Australia: Index Mundi. Retrieved May 6, 2013, from http://www.indexmundi.com/australia/infant_mortality_rate.html

Australian Institute of Health and Welfare (AIHW). (2013a). *National health priority areas.* Canberra: Australian Government. Retrieved May 18, 2013, from http:// www.aihw.gov.au/national-health-priority-areas/

——. (2013b). *Health workforce.* Canberra: Australian Government. Retrieved May 9, 2013, from http://www.aihw.gov.au/health-workforce/

Australian Nursing and Midwifery Accreditation Council (ANMAC). (2010). About ANMAC. Retrieved May 6, 2013, from http://www.anmac.org.au/about-anmac

Commonwealth Fund. (2013). *The health care system and health policy in Australia.* New York: Commonwealth Fund. Retrieved May 7, 2013, from http://www. commonwealthfund.org/Fellowships/Australian-American-Health-Policy-Fellowships/The-Health-Care-System-And-Health-Policy-In-Australia.Aspx

Department of Families, Housing, Community Services & Indigenous Affairs. (2013). Closing the gap. Canberra: Australian Government. Retrieved May 6, 2013, from http://www.fahcsia.gov.au/our-responsibilities/indigenous-australians/ programs-services/closing-the-gap

Francis, K., Chapman, Y., Hoare, K. & Birks, M. (2013). The Australian healthcare system. In K. Francis, Y. Chapman, K. Hoare & M. Birks (Eds.), *Australia and New Zealand, community as partner: Theory and practice in nursing* (Chapter 3) (2nd ed.). Sydney: Wolters Kluwer/Lippincott, Williams and Wilkins.

Harvey, N. & Park, T. (2011). Cultures and nursing. In A.Berman et al. (Eds.), *Kozier and Erb's fundamentals of nursing* (Chapter 19) (2nd ed.). Frenchs Forest, NSW: Pearson Australia.

Health Workforce Australia (HWA). (2012a). *Health workforce 2025 – Doctors, Nurses and Midwives* – Volume 1. Adelaide: HWA. Retrieved May 15, 2013, from http://www.hwa.gov.au/sites/uploads/health-workforce-2025-volume-1.pdf

———. (2012b). *Health workforce 2025 – Doctors, Nurses and Midwives* – Volume 2. Adelaide: HWA. Retrieved May 15, 2013, from http://www.hwa.gov.au/sites/uploads/HW2025Volume2_FINAL-20120424.pdf

———. (2013). About us. Adelaide: Australian Government. Retrieved May 15, 2013, from http://www.hwa.gov.au/about

Indigenous Allied Health Australia (AIHA). (2013). *Improving cultural responsiveness of health professionals through education reform*. Canberra: IAHA Secretariat.

Indigenous Australia. (2013). *Aboriginal kinship and families*. Indigenous Australia. Retrieved May 6, 2013, from http://www.indigenousaustralia.info/social-structure/kinship.html

Morrisey, C. (1924, February 16). La Perouse. His share in Australian history. *The Sydney Morning Herald*. Retrieved May 6, 2013, from http://trove.nla.gov.au/ndp/del/article/16123564

Museum of New Zealand Te Papa Tongarewa. (2013). The Endeavour and Captain Cook's first voyage (25 Aug 1768–12 Jul 1771). New Zealand: Museum of New Zealand Te Papa Tongarewa. Retrieved May 6, 2013, from http://collections.tepapa.govt.nz/theme.aspx?irn=572

Olila, E. (2005). Global health priorities – priorities of the wealthy? *Global Health*, 1(6). doi: 10.1186/1744-8603-1-6. Retrieved May 18, 2013, from http://www.ncbi.nlm.nih.gov/pmc/articles/PMC1143784/

Podger, A. & Hagan, P. (1999). *Reforming the Australian health care system, the role of government*. Canberra: DoHA. Retrieved May 6, 2013, from: http://www.health.gov.au/internet/main/publishing.nsf/Content/545A13C576C6DE24CA2574860013D93A/$File/ocpanew1.pdf

Tourism Australia. (2013a). Australia's culture. Canberra: Tourism Australia. Retrieved May 6, 2013, from http://www.australia.com/about/culture-history/culture.aspx

———. (2013b). Australia's history. Canberra: Tourism Australia. Retrieved May 6, 2013, from http://www.australia.com/about/culture-history/history.aspx

2 Rural health

Desley Hegney, Karen Francis and Jane Mills

Learning objectives On completion of this chapter, the reader will be able to:

- define 'rurality'

- describe rural and remote Australia as a place to live and work, highlighting recent changes in the economic, social and industrial fabric of rural and remote communities that impact on health

- recognise the importance of rural and remote area nursing within the rural health workforce

- identify the advantages and disadvantages of rural and remote area nursing and midwifery

- create a resource bank of references and web links for readers to use in further exploring rural and remote area nursing in Australia.

Key words Rurality, rural health, health workforce, rural nursing and midwifery, health status

Chapter overview

This chapter contextualises 'rurality' as a criterion for classifying populations living in areas outside major cities. Differences in health status of rural compared to metropolitan communities are described, as is the composition of the health workforce. The chapter concludes with an overview of the rural nursing and midwifery workforce and the challenges these clinicians face in the delivery of care.

Introduction

Approximately 31% of the Australian population live outside major cities (e.g. capital cities or large regional centres with populations over 250 000). Only about 2% of this rural population live in what are considered to be 'remote' communities (Australian Institute of Health and Welfare [AIHW], 2012a). The percentage of the Australian population living in rural areas has declined considerably over the two centuries of white settlement. Much of this attrition has been caused by the merging of family farms (agribusiness) and young farmers leaving 'the land' to work and live in major centres (Smith, 2007). The economics of agriculture (e.g. the strong Australian dollar) and the increasing regulation of the industry have meant that the rural population has declined. Further, those still working in the agricultural sector represent an ageing workforce. This population decline and the ageing of the agricultural workforce have been a continuous feature of rural Australia and have occurred not only in livestock and grain industries but also in the fruit and vegetable industry (Smith, 2007; Sutherland, 2012).

Agriculture, however, represents only one industry in rural and remote Australia. Other key industries include mining, forestry and fishing. All of these industries are considered to have high occupational risks and contribute to the differences in morbidity and mortality rates in rural and remote communities (Smith, 2007).

Definition

An array of classification systems has been developed to isolate and describe 'rural' environments, including the Accessibility Remoteness Index of Australia (ARIA), the Rural Remote Metropolitan Access classification (RRMA) and the Griffith Service Access Frame (GSAF) (Francis, Chapman, Hoare & Birks, 2013). Many classification systems define rural in terms of non-metropolitan or non-urban, while others base their definitions on population in relationship to geographical distance (e.g. square kilometres) and/or distance from specific services and usage of land (e.g. agriculture) (U.S. Department of Health and Human Services, 2013). Australia has traditionally based the various classification systems on population density versus landmass (Baxter, Hayes & Gray, 2011; Commonwealth of Australia, 2012).

Currently, healthcare services in Australia use the ARIA, which was revised and is now known as the ARIA+. This version is inclusive of more information on the location of service centres. This system has six classifications that relate to the ARIA+ calculation for each census collection district (CCD) and are presented in Table 2.1 (Australian Bureau of Statistics [ABS], 2011b).

TABLE 2.1 *Remoteness area and ARIA+ values.*

REMOTENESS AREA NAME	CCD AVERAGE ARIA+ VALUE RANGES
Major Cities of Australia	0 to 0.2
Inner Regional Australia	greater than 0.2 and less than or equal to 2.4
Outer Regional Australia	greater than 2.4 and less than or equal to 5.92
Remote Australia	greater than 5.92 and less than or equal to 10.53
Very Remote Australia	greater than 10.53
Migratory	off-shore, migratory and shipping CCDs

Source: ABS (2011). *Remoteness Structure*

Rural communities

Rurality is often equated with an idyllic way of life: rolling plains, sunshine, a slower pace of life, better health and improved life chances (AIHW, 2008; Smith, 2007; Humphreys & Rolley, 1991). There is also the Australian 'myth' of the stoic bushman working hard, struggling to make ends meet (being a 'battler') supported by his hardworking wife. The stoicism of the Australian rural person has been linked to their health status, that is, carrying on despite illness and injury and not being one to demand or complain (AIHW, 2004; Land and Water Australia, 2004; Lovett, 1993; Walmsley & Sorensen, 1988). Australian rural and remote populations are very diverse however, and in the 21st century this image of rural battlers sits side by side with the image of the 'fly-in'/'fly-out' (FIFO) workers. FIFO workers are mainly utilised by mining companies in Western Australia and Queensland and live in self-contained accommodation (see Chapter 7). While this group draws on community services (health in particular), the workers are not seen as an integral part of the community as their families live outside the mining town.

In addition to this extra demand on rural and remote health services by FIFO workers, transient retirees commonly known as 'grey-haired nomads' create a further demand. This group consists, in the main, of people over the age of 50 years. They travel around Australia using a car and caravan (or reticulated vehicle) and, particularly during the peak tourist periods (e.g. winter time in northern Australia), can double or triple the population of small rural and remote communities overnight. As many small health services are staffed to meet the demand of off-season population densities, 'grey nomads' with chronic diseases and comorbidities cause unforeseen pressure on resources, including nurses (Tate, Mein, Freeman & Maguire, 2006).

Research over many years has demonstrated that rural populations have considerably different mortality and morbidity rates from those living in major cities. For example, rural people are more likely to have chronic conditions (diabetes, cancer, depression, arthritis), poorer dental health, more motor vehicle accidents and a higher suicide rate (AIHW, 2008, 2010; Smith, 2007; Smith, Humphreys & Wilson, 2008).

Many of these health states are a result of the lower socioeconomic status of rural people and the difficulty they face (in expense and time) in accessing health services. While some large rural hospitals provide limited specialist services (such as chemotherapy), many rural people have to travel to obtain radiotherapy and general and specialised surgery. The cost of travel and accommodation and the loss of income may mean that some people may choose not to seek specialist treatment even though all Australian states and territories provide travel and accommodation subsidies (ABS, 2013a). Hegney, Pearce, Rogers-Clark and Martin-McDonald (2005) found that, faced with travel and loss of income for radiotherapy, some rural people chose not to have treatment. Obviously, access is a major causative factor in the health inequities of rural people (AIHW, 2013).

Health and healthcare service provision in rural contexts

As highlighted previously (see Chapter 1), rural communities are generally defined according to the density of population versus landmass (which are inversely proportional) – that is, the greater the landmass, the smaller the population. The population in Australia decreases the greater the distance from coastal areas, specifically from the capital cities of each state and territory (ABS, 2013b). This settlement pattern has resulted in the highest concentration of health and other services being located in areas of high population. People who live in rural and remote settings therefore have less access to the range of services that urban populations take for granted. As the population becomes less dense, the range of services also decreases, and those that are available are more generalist than specialist in nature (AIHW, 2013).

Rural and remote nurses and midwives

Nurses are the largest group of health professionals nationally and the most highly represented in the rural setting (AIHW, 2012b). Health Workforce Australia (HWA) (2012a) asserts that while nurses are the most constant of the health professional groups in rural and remote settings, nursing shortages are growing, and they predict that health outcomes will be compromised if this phenomenon is not addressed. The majority of rural midwives are also nurses (see Chapter 4) and often work as both nurses and midwives, particularly in health facilities that are not regional centres (Francis & Mills, 2011; HWA, 2012b).

In remote areas, nurses work in posts where they provide health services to their community in conjunction with Aboriginal and Torres Strait Islander healthcare workers (Kruske et al., 2013). These nurses lead primary care teams that are often part of a 'hub and spoke' model, which specialist services (e.g. doctors, specialist nurses, diabetes educators, social workers and psychologists) visit on a regular basis.

As the population density increases, remote nursing clinics are replaced by small rural hospitals. Nurses staff small rural hospitals, often with the assistance of a general practitioner (GP) in private practice (Mills, Birks & Hegney, 2010) who provides a visiting service (HWA, 2012a; Sullivan, Francis & Hegney, 2008, 2010; Sullivan, Hegney & Francis, 2012). The number of beds in a small rural hospital varies. Most rural hospitals would have aged care residents in either a hospital bed or a freestanding facility within the grounds.

Rural nurses are also required to deal with the many unplanned visits to the hospital by those seeking emergency care (Mills et al., 2010; Sullivan et al., 2010). As there is normally no dedicated emergency department, the nurse leaves the general ward to attend to the emergency (Sullivan, 2013). In severe cases, a person may be brought in by ambulance and the doctor alerted. In less severe cases, the nurse will deal with the case.

Similar to remote area health services, both hospital and community rural health services usually rely on a 'hub and spoke' model for visiting specialist services. Video-enabled specialist services known as telehealth, e-health, m-health (mobile health devices) or telemedicine provide both opportunities and challenges (Sabesan et al., 2012). Both rural and remote nurses are instrumental in the provision of telehealth services as they are often the intermediary between the patient and the videoconferenced specialist service (Ellis, 2004;

Sabesan et al., 2012). While there is evidence that video-enabled specialist services are effective, access to information technology can be varied across Australia. A study of nurses' usage of information technology found that rural nurses had less access to information technology than remote area nurses. The latter not only used information systems to support their care but also had better access to the intranet and the internet (Eley, Fallon, Soar, Buikstra & Hegney, 2008). Many health services now regularly use videoconferencing for education, networking and patient consultation (Boots, Singh & Lipman, 2012; Gray, Armfield & Smith, 2010; Sabesan et al., 2012).

Models of care

There are several generalist specialist models of rural and remote area nursing practice being used in Australia. In Queensland and Victoria, for example, there is a scheduled medicines endorsed advanced nursing practice model (Hegney, McKeon, Plank, Raith & Watson, 2003; Sullivan, 2013). This model is known as the Rural and Isolated Practice Endorsed Registered Nurse (RIPERN) (Department of Health Victoria, 2013). There are five aspects of this program:

1 evidence-based clinical guidelines known as the Primary Clinical Care Manual (PCCM) (Fry, Borg, Jackson & McAlpine, 1999; Latter & Courtenay, 2004; MacLeod & Zimmer, 2005; Sullivan et al., 2008; Woods, 1999)

2 a nationally accredited program of education that leads to an endorsement to practise in this advanced practice role and to supply scheduled medicines (Bradley & Nolan, 2007; Hegney et al., 2003; Sullivan, 2013; Webb & Gibson, 2011)

3 drugs that nurses can administer and supply in accordance with the PCCM as per the Queensland Drug Therapy Protocol or the Victorian Minister for Health's Gazetted Approval (MacLeod & Zimmer, 2005; Stewart, Stansfield & Tapp, 2004; Webb & Gibson, 2011)

4 a list of health facilities or areas where nurses can work in this role (this includes the flight nurses when working on a Royal Flying Doctor Service (RFDS) plane in Queensland), and

5 the legislation and change management to support this (changes to the Queensland Health [Drugs and Poisons] Act and Regulations, and the Victorian Drugs, Poisons and Controlled Substances Act and Regulations) (Cipher, Hooker & Guerra, 2006; Cooper et al., 2011; Dehn & Day, 2007; Dewar & Sharp, 2006; McCormack & Garbett, 2003; Murphy, Martin-Misener, Cooke & Sketris, 2009; Rogers, 2003).

The principal outcome of the model is to improve community access to evidence-based primary and emergency care. The RIPERN model was adopted in both Queensland and Victoria to enhance the resilience of rural and isolated health service delivery, particularly in the face of workforce shortages. The RIPERN model provides a coherent legislative and clinical risk management framework within which registered nurses are enabled to practise at a more advanced, autonomous level consistently. As a generalist specialist model, the RIPERN role supplements and complements the roles of existing health professionals and can provide a clinical career pathway between the registered nurse and nurse practitioner. As a result of national registration and regulation, the standards for an endorsed scheduled medicine endorsement are currently under review. It is possible that the ability of nurses to administer and supply medications from evidence-based protocols will be expanded from rural and remote to other settings.

The other model of generalist specialist nursing practice in rural and remote areas is that of the nurse practitioner. Initially designed to provide care to rural and remote residents, Australian nurse practitioners are largely based in metropolitan health services, with a number employed in rural services (particularly in the emergency departments of public hospitals).

The roles of rural and remote area nurses are similar. The remote area nurse, as mentioned earlier, is normally the sole registered nurse in their community (Kruske et al., 2013), usually working with Aboriginal and Torres Strait Islander healthcare workers (Coyle, Al-Motlaq, Mills, Francis & Birks, 2010). In the main, these nurses provide primary care, respond to emergencies and manage community members presenting to their clinic with a range of healthcare issues. They also provide a primary healthcare service to the community, but the emphasis placed on preventative care in this role is variable across the country (Birks et al., 2010). Remote area nurses are reliant on an off-site medical practitioner who is contactable by telephone or via the RFDS, and therefore these nurses require advanced assessment and management skills (Francis & Jacob, 2011; Kruske et al., 2013). This is particularly important in emergency situations where they may wait several hours for an aircraft to come to their assistance (Kruske et al., 2013).

A major benefit of rural and remote nursing practice is the ability to work in an autonomous but collaborative manner (Cooper, O'Carroll, Jenkin & Badger, 2007; Skår, 2009; Sullivan, 2013). Nurses who move into rural and remote nursing practice or provide locum or relief services (Becker, McCutcheon & Hegney, 2010) often find the broad scope and lack of on-site health professionals challenging. However, those who choose to permanently work as a rural or remote area nurse find this aspect of practice rewarding (Mills et al., 2010). Because permanent rural and remote nurses and nurse/midwives live and work in the same community in a generalist specialist role, they are often referred to as providing 'womb to tomb' care (Hegney, 1997, 1998; Mills et al., 2010). Nursing care in these roles ranges across the lifespan. Knowing the person to whom care is delivered can have its advantages and disadvantages (Hegney, 1996b). In rural communities, nurses tend to remain in one position for long periods of time, with turnover occurring only when, for example, a nurse moves from working in a hospital to working for a GP. In other words, nurses do not leave nursing, they just change their employer (Hegney, McCarthy, Rogers-Clark & Gorman, 2002). This contrasts with the higher turnover of staff in remote nursing posts, due mostly to long on-call hours and the challenging nature of working in remote communities (Kruske et al., 2013).

Challenges

While there are many advantages of being a rural and remote nurse, there are also challenges to be faced. Some of these challenges include the following.

Being known within the community

Rural and remote area nurses are highly visible members of the community (McConnell-Henry, Chapman & Francis, 2010). While a higher turnover of nurses in remote communities is more likely, rural nurses usually have strong ties with their community (Mills et al., 2010). For example, they may be a property owner or a partner in a business. Their children go to the local school, and in some instances their families have been in the area for several generations. Therefore, when the rural nurse is caring for a person, there is an added pressure for confidentiality (Hegney, 1996a; Mills et al., 2010). Additionally, there is the constant feeling of never being off duty. It is not uncommon for rural residents to seek out the nurse first – in the supermarket, walking down the street – before seeking a medical practitioner's assistance (see Chapter 4). Some nurses find this the most difficult part of rural nursing (Hegney, 1996a; McConnell-Henry et al., 2010; Mills et al., 2010). These challenges are further discussed in Chapter 3.

Mentoring

Identifying a mentor when nurses move to a rural or remote location is an important strategy to increase both local knowledge and personal resilience. There are three areas that new or novice rural or remote nurses need mentoring in: culture, politics and clinical practice (Mills, Francis & Bonner, 2007b). Finding the right person to be a mentor can be challenging, but achieving this goal can be professionally rewarding. Mentoring relationships can occur as a result of a new or novice rural or remote nurse experiencing a critical incident, leading them to turn to a more experienced colleague for guidance and support. This type of supportive relationship can be short term – in which case it can be termed 'accidental mentoring' (Mills, Francis & Bonner, 2007a). Other types of mentoring relationships that are longer term develop as a result of a formal continuing professional program or serendipitously because two people share the same values and beliefs. As the new or novice rural or remote nurse and their more experienced counterpart spend time together, levels of trust and engagement grow, resulting in them getting to know the stranger who is now their mentor (Mills, Francis & Bonner, 2008).

Adequate preparation for rural and remote nursing practice

It is clear that rural and remote nursing practice is quite different from practice in larger centres. Over the past decade, several research studies have been carried out on what constitutes adequate preparation for the role, from both a clinical and a cultural perspective (Kenny, Carter, Martin & Williams, 2004; Kruske et al., 2013; Lea & Cruickshank, 2007). Other studies have examined what attracts student nurses to work in a rural environment (Lea et al., 2008). All agree that the preparation provided in entry-to-practice programs influences choices to work in rural nursing and also the ability of the novice rural or remote area nurse to practise in a competent manner. Additionally, being culturally responsive is essential requirement for all practitioners and should be used as an overarching principle when working with all facets of the community (Kruske et al., 2013). However, having an understanding of history and the impact for Aboriginal and Torres Strait Islander people within the context of contemporary Aboriginal and Torres Strait Islander lives is crucial to delivering culturally responsive care.

Accessing continual professional education

Under national legislation, nurses must complete a minimum of 20 hours of continuing professional development per annum. While there has been some improvement in accessibility to continuing education (mostly due to the flexible way that continuing professional development is delivered), time and cost continue to be the major barriers to rural and remote area nurses' ability to meet their mandatory learning target (Hegney, 1997; Mills et al., 2010). The role of rural nurses and midwives is further examined in Chapter 4.

Tracey is a rural student nurse who has been assigned to a small rural community healthcare team in New South Wales for her community placement. Elaine, who has been a community nurse for 25 years, is mentoring her. Elaine asks Tracey to help her prepare for a Men's Health evening in which Elaine will talk about common complaints for men in rural areas.

VIGNETTE

Questions
1   What might be some of the health issues Tracey may suggest to Elaine to discuss?
2   How will Tracey ensure Elaine has the most up-to-date information?
     The evening commences with Elaine giving an overview of what will be discussed. During the presentation, Tracey notices that a gentleman in the audience seems to be anxious and distressed.
3   What action should Tracey take?
4   How will Tracey maintain confidentiality and respect for this man?
     On closer discussion with the man, Tracey identifies that he is called Bob and he is a distant relative of hers. He is a second cousin of her mother and they had lost touch for many years.
5   Will Tracey inform her mother that she has met Bob?
6   How will she establish communication between Bob and her mother?
     Bob lives alone. He has never married and is an active member of the community. On Tracey's last day of practicum, she and Elaine have to make a visit to Bob as he has received some bad news from his recent blood tests. It seems Bob has early prostate cancer and he wants to know what to do next.
7   What responses might Elaine give to Bob?
8   What role should Tracey assume in this interaction?

Summary

Populations that reside in rural and remote communities have differential access to health and other services compared to urban counterparts.

In this chapter, we have:

- defined classifications of rurality and remoteness
- highlighted the variability of rural and remote contexts
- described rural populations
- provided details of the health workforce
- discussed models of care utilised.

Reflective questions

1 What differences do you see in nursing roles as the decreasing populations in rural areas make the employment of other health professionals unsustainable? What opportunities are there for rural and remote area nurses?
2 How can nurses best use e-health and m-health (mobile health devices) in the prevention and treatment of illness and injury?
3 Given the growing multicultural mix of rural and remote communities, what is the best model for cultural awareness preparation for rural and remote area nurses?
4 What are the opportunities for extending a scheduled medicines and nurse practitioner model in rural and remote communities?
5 How would this initiative link for a clinical career pathway?
6 How can we best support rural and remote area nurses once they are in practice?

Useful websites

Australian College of Nursing
http://www.acn.edu.au

Australian Government – Department of Health, Rural and Regional Health Australia
http://www.ruralhealthaustralia.gov.au/internet/rha/Publishing.nsf/Content/Publications

Australian Institute of Health and Welfare
http://www.aihw.gov.au

CRANAplus
https://crana.org.au/

Health Workforce Australia
http://www.hwa.gov.au

National Rural Health Alliance
http://www.ruralhealth.org.au

Rural Classifications
http://www.ruralhealthaustralia.gov.au/internet/rha/publishing.nsf/Content/locator

References

Australian Bureau of Statistic (ABS). (2011). *Remoteness structure*. Retrieved January 3, 2012, from http://www.abs.gov.au/websitedbs/D3310114.nsf/home/remoteness+structure

——. (2013a). *1301.0 – Year Book Australia, 2012*. Retrieved May 6, 2013, from http://www.abs.gov.au/ausstats/abs@.nsf/Lookup/by Subject/1301.0~2012~Main Features~Australia's climate~143

——. (2013b). Population, 2013. Retrieved May 6, 2013, from http://www.abs.gov. au/ausstats/abs@.nsf/Lookup/by Subject/1370.0~2010~Chapter~Population distribution (3.3)

Australian Institute of Health and Welfare (AIHW). (2004). *Rural, regional and remote health: A study on mortality*. Canberra:Australian Government.

——. (2008). *Australia's health*. Canberra: AIHW.

——. (2010). *Australia's health 2010*. Health series no. 12. Cat no. AUS 122. Canberra: AIHW.

——. (2012a). *Australia's health 2012* (Vol. 2013). Canberra: AIHW.

——. (2012b). *Nursing and midwifery workforce 2011*. Canberra: AIHW.

——. (2013). Rural health. Retrieved September 8, 2013, from http://www.aihw.gov. au/rural-health/

Baxter, J., Hayes, A. & Gray, M. (2011). Families in regional, rural and remote Australia [Factsheet]. Melbourne: Australian Institute of Family Studies. Retrieved September 30, 2013, from http://www.aifs.gov.au/institute/pubs/ factssheets/2011/fs201103.html

Becker, S., McCutcheon, H. & Hegney, D. (2010). Casualisation in the nursing workforce – the need to make it work. *Australian Journal of Advanced Nursing*, 28(1), 45–51.

Birks, M., Mills, J., Francis, K., Coyle, M., Davis, J. & Jones, J. (2010). Models of health service delivery in remote or isolated areas of Queensland: A multiple case study. *Australian Journal of Advanced Nursing*, 28(1), 25–34. Retrieved March 24, 2014, from http://www.ajan.com.au/Vol28/28-1_Birks.pdf

Boots, R. J., Singh, S. J. & Lipman, J. (2012). The tyranny of distance: Telemedicine for the critically ill in rural Australia. *Anaesthesia and Intensive Care*, 40(5), 871–4.

Bradley, E. & Nolan, P. (2007). Impact of nurse prescribing: A qualitative study. *Journal of Advanced Nursing*, 59(2), 120–8. doi: 10.1111/j.1365–2648.2007.04295.x

Cipher, D. J., Hooker, R. S. & Guerra, P. (2006). Prescribing trends by nurse practitioners and physician assistants in the United States. *Journal of the American Academy of Nurse Practitioners*, 18(6), 291–6. doi: 10.1111/j.1745–7599.2006.00133.x

Commonwealth of Australia. (2012). *National Strategic Framework for Rural and Remote Health*. Endorsed by the Standing Council on Health, 11 November 2011. Canberra: Australian Government. Retrieved March 24, 2014, from http://www. ruralhealthaustralia.gov.au/internet/rha/publishing.nsf/Content/EBD8D28B517 296A3CA2579FF000350C6/$File/NationalStrategicFramework.pdf

Cooper, R. J., Bissell, P., Ward, P., Murphy, E., Anderson, C., Avery, T., … Ratcliffe, J. (2011). Further challenges to medical dominance? The case of nurse and pharmacist supplementary prescribing. *Health*, 16(2), 115–33. doi: 10.1177/1363459310364159

Cooper, S., O'Carroll, J., Jenkin, A. & Badger, B. (2007). Collaborative practices in unscheduled emergency care: Role and impact of the emergency care practitioner – qualitative and summative findings. *Emergency Medicine Journal*, 24(9), 625.

Coyle, M., Al-Motlaq, M. A., Mills, J., Francis, K. & Birks, M. (2010). An integrative review of the role of registered nurses in remote and isolated practice. *Australian Health Review*, 34(2), 239–45.

Dehn, M. & Day, G. (2007). Managing in an increasingly complex health care environment: Perceptions of Queensland hospital managers. *Asia Pacific Journal of Health Management*, 2(3), 30–6.

Department of Health Victoria. (2013). Rural and isolated practice endorsed registered nurse. Retrieved September 8, 2013, from http://health.vic.gov.au/ruralhealth/ripern/index.htm

Dewar, B. & Sharp, C. (2006). Using evidence: How action learning can support individual and organisational learning through action research. *Educational Action Research*, 14(2), 219–37.

Eley, R., Fallon, T., Soar, J., Buikstra, E. & Hegney, D. (2008). Barriers to use of information and computer technology by Australia's nurses: A national survey. *Journal of Clinical Nursing*, 18(8), 1151–8. doi: 10.1111/j.1365–2702.2008.02336.x

Ellis, I. (2004). Is telehealth the right tool for remote communities? Improving health status in rural Australia. *Contemporary Nurse*, 16(3), 163–8.

Francis, K., Chapman, Y., Hoare, K. & Birks, M. (2013). Promoting healthy partnerships with rural populations. In K. Francis, Y. Chapman, K. Hoare & M. Birks (Eds.), *Australia and New Zealand, community as partner, theory and practice in nursing* (pp. 372–85). Sydney: Wolters Kluwer, Lippincott, Williams & Wilkins.

Francis, K. & Jacob, E. (2011). Rural nursing in the Australian context. In D. Molinari & A. Bushy (Eds.), *The rural nurse: Transition to practice* (pp. 95–108). New York: Springer.

Francis, K. L. & Mills, J. E. (2011). Sustaining and growing the rural nursing and midwifery workforce: Understanding the issues and isolating directions for the future. *Collegian*, 18(2), 55–60. doi: 10.1016/j.colegn.2010.08.003

Fry, M., Borg, A., Jackson, S. & McAlpine, A. (1999). The advanced clinical nurse a new model of practice: Meeting the challenge of peak activity periods. *Australasian Emergency Nursing Journal*, 2(3), 26–8.

Gray, L. C., Armfield, N. R. & Smith, A. C. (2010). Telemedicine for wound care: Current practice and future potential. *Wound Practice and Research* 18(4), 158–63.

Health Workforce Australia (HWA). (2012a). *Health Workforce 2025 – Doctors, Nurses and Midwives – Volume 1*. Adelaide: Health Workforce Australia.

——. (2012b). *Health Workforce 2025 – Doctors, Nurses and Midwives – Volume 2*. Adelaide: Health Workforce Australia.

Hegney, D. (1996a). The status of rural nursing in Australia: A review. *Australian Journal of Rural Health*, 4, 1–10.

——. (1996b). The windmill of rural health: A foucauldian analysis of the discourses of rural nursing in Australia, 1991–1994 (Unpublished PhD thesis). Southern Cross University.

——. (1997). Rural nursing practice. In L.Siegloff (Ed.), *Rural nursing in the Australian context* (pp. 25–44). Canberra: Royal College of Nursing Australia.

——. (1998). The advanced practice role of the rural nurse: Challenging the culture of nursing, pharmacy and medicine. Paper presented at the Cultures in Caring, 4th Biennial Australian Rural and Remote Health Scientific Conference, Toowoomba, Qld.

Hegney, D., McCarthy, A., Rogers-Clark, C. & Gorman, D. (2002). Factors affecting the retention of the rural and remote area nursing workforce in Queensland, Australia. *The Journal of Nursing Administration*, 32(3), 128–35.

Hegney, D., McKeon, C., Plank, A., Raith, L. & Watson, J. (2003). *The administration and supply of controlled and restricted medications by Queensland rural and remote nurses*. Brisbane: Queensland Nursing Council.

Hegney, D., Pearce, S., Rogers-Clark, C. & Martin-McDonald, K. (2005). Close, but still too far. The experiences of people with cancer commuting from a provincial town to a major city for radiotherapy treatment. *European Journal of Cancer Care*, 14, 75–82.

Humphreys, J. S. & Rolley, F. (1991). *Health and health care in rural Australia. A literature review*. Armidale: University of New England, Armidale.

Kenny, A., Carter, L., Martin, S. & Williams, S. (2004). Why four years when three will do? Enhanced knowledge for rural practice. *Nursing Inquiry*, 11, 108–16.

Kruske, S., Lenthall, S., Kildea, S., Knight, S., MacKay, B. & Hegney, D. (2013). Rural and remote area nursing. In D. Brown & H. Edwards (Eds.), *Lewis's Medical-Surgical Nursing* (4th ed.). Marrickville, NSW: Elsevier Australia.

Land and Water Australia. (2004). *Australia's farmers: Past, present and future*. Canberra: Australian Government

Latter, S. & Courtenay, M. (2004). Effectiveness of nurse prescribing: A review of the literature. *Journal of Clinical Nursing*, 13(1), 26–32. doi: 10.1046/j.1365–2702.2003.00839.x

Lea, J. & Cruickshank, M. (2007). The experience of new graduate nurses in rural practice in New South Wales. *Rural and Remote Health*, 7(814), (Online).

Lea, J., Cruickshank, M., Paliadelis, P., Parmenter, G., Sanderson, H. & Thornberry, P. (2008). The lure of the bush: Do rural placements influence student nurses to seek employment in rural settings? *Collegian*, 15, 77–82.

Lovett, J. (1993). Foreword. In T. Sorensen & R. Epps (Eds.), *Prospects and policies for rural Australia* (pp. vii–ix). Melbourne: Longman Cheshire.

MacLeod, M. & Zimmer, L. (2005). Rethinking emancipation and empowerment in action research: Lessons from small rural hospitals. *The Canadian Journal of Nursing Research*, 37(1), 68–84.

McConnell-Henry, T., Chapman, Y. & Francis, K. (2010). Rural nursing: Looking after people we know. *Australian Nursing Journal*, 17(8), 42.

McCormack, B. & Garbett, R. (2003). The characteristics, qualities and skills of practice developers. *Journal of Clincial Nursing*, 12, 317–25.

Mills, J., Birks, M. & Hegney, D. (2010). The status of rural nursing in Australia: 12 years on. *Collegian*, 17(1), 30–7. doi: 10.1016/j.colegn.2009.09.001

Mills, J., Francis, K. & Bonner, A. (2007a). The accidental mentor: Australian rural nurses developing supportive relationships in the workplace. *Rural and Remote Health*, 7(842), (Online).

——. (2007b). Live my work: Rural nurses and their multiple perspectives of self. *Journal of Advanced Nursing*, 59(6), 583–90. doi: 10.1111/j.1365–2648.2007.04350.x

——. (2008). Getting to know a stranger – rural nurses' experiences of mentoring: A grounded theory. *International Journal of Nursing Studies*, 45(4), 599–607. doi: 10.1016/j.ijnurstu.2006.12.003

Murphy, A., Martin-Misener, R., Cooke, C. & Sketris, I. (2009). Administrative claims data analysis of nurse practitioner prescribing for older adults. *Journal of Advanced Nursing*, 65(10), 2077–87. doi: 10.1111/j.1365–2648.2009.05069.x

Rogers, E. M. (2003). *Diffusion of innovations* (5th ed.). New York: Free Press.

Sabesan, S., Larkins, S., Varma, S., Andrews, A., Beuttner, P., Brennan, S. & Young, M. (2012). Telemedicine for rural cancer care in North Queensland: Bringing cancer care home. *Australian Journal of Rural Health*, 20(5), 259–64.

Skår, R. (2009). The meaning of autonomy in nursing practice. *Journal of Clinical Nursing*, 19, 2226–34.

Smith, J. D. (2007). Rural people's health. In J. D.Smith (Ed.), *Australia's rural and remote health: A social justice perspective* (2nd ed.), (pp. 121–33). Croydon, Vic: Tertiary Press.

Smith, K. B., Humphreys, J. S. & Wilson, M. G. A. (2008). Addressing the health disadvantage of rural populations: How does epidemiological evidence inform rural health policies and research? *Australian Journal of Rural Health*, 16, 56–66.

Stewart, J., Stansfield, K. & Tapp, D. (2004). Clinical nurses' understanding of autonomy. *The Journal of Nursing Administration*, 34(10), 443–50.

Sullivan, E. (2013). 'All Hands on Deck' – An autonomous collaborative practice model to sustain emergency care in rural Victoria. (PhD thesis, Monash University, Melbourne). Retrieved March 24, 2014, from http://arrow.monash.edu.au/hdl/1959.1/814243

Sullivan, E., Francis, K. & Hegney, D. (2008). Review of small rural health services in Victoria: How does the nursing–medical division of labour affect access to emergency care? *Journal of Clinical Nursing*, 17(12), 1543–52. doi: 10.1111/j.1365–2702.2007.02087.x

———. (2010). Triage, treat and transfer: Reconceptualising a rural practice model. *Journal of Clinical Nursing*, 19(11–12), 1625–34. doi: 10.1111/j.1365-2702.2009.03073.x

Sullivan, E., Hegney, D. & Francis, K. (2012). Victorian rural emergency care – a case for advancing nursing practice. *International Journal of Nursing Practice*, 18(3), 226–32.

Sutherland, K. (2012). Ageing agricultural workforce concern. Retrieved March 24, 2014, from http://www.stockjournal.com.au/news/agriculture/agribusiness/general-news/ageing-agricultural-workforce-concern/2627116.aspx

Tate, J., Mein, J., Freeman, H. & Maguire, G. (2006). Grey nomads – health and health preparation of older travellers in remote Australia. *Australian Farm Physician*, 35(1–2), 70–2.

U. S. Department of Health and Human Services. (2013). How is rural defined? Retrieved July 8, 2013, from http://www.hrsa.gov/healthit/toolbox/RuralHealthITtoolbox/Introduction/defined.html

Walmsley, D. & Sorensen, A. (1988). *Contemporary Australia*. Melbourne: Longman Cheshire.

Webb, W. A. & Gibson, V. (2011). Evaluating the impact of nurse independent prescribing in a weekend clinical nurse specialist service. *International Journal of Palliative Nursing*, 17(11), 537–43.

Woods, L. (1999). The contingent nature of advanced nursing practice. *Journal of Advanced Nursing*, 30(1), 121–8. doi: 10.1046/j.1365-2648.1999.01055.x

3 Understanding the community

Ysanne Chapman, Karen Francis and Melanie Birks

Learning objectives On completion of this chapter, the reader will be able to:

- describe the features of a community profile and identify sources of data to inform this process

- critically examine issues of access and equity in respect of health services

- identify the information needed to inform prospective community planning

- discuss the concept of burden of disease

- appreciate the impact of contemporary communication systems on health outcomes.

Key words Burden of disease, community profile, rural communities, rural nursing, midwifery

Chapter overview

Working effectively in any community requires understanding of the community. Such an understanding can be obtained through knowing the population demographics, resources and assets of that community. Together, these features make up a community profile that forms the basis for planning to address the burden of disease and inequity in health outcomes and accessibility to services in rural and remote areas. This chapter provides details of methods for building a community profile in which rural nurses and midwives work.

Community profile

A community profile is a summary of the community that is inclusive of the population, assets, resources and trends (social, political and economic)

that provide baseline data (Australian Bureau of Statistics [ABS], 2013b). These data provide the context for determining need, planning and assessing the impact of proposed initiatives (New Forest District Council, 2013). The community profile is harnessed by drawing on primary data that are generated through observations, stakeholder interviews, surveys, an inventory of services and facilities, and secondary data sources such as reports produced by local councils, businesses, the ABS census, workforce/labour and housing data, newspapers and other media communications (*Community profiling*, 2004; New Forest District Council, 2013). These data must be collated in a manner that is informative and useful. Developing community profiles is an iterative process that allows for new information to be included as it is isolated (Francis, Chapman, Hoare & Birks, 2013).

Demographic profile

When developing a community profile, it is necessary to know about the population that resides in the community (*Community profiling*, 2004). Information on population demographics can be accessed via the ABS (2013a). Characteristics of the population such as age, ethnicity, gender, income, migration, employment and unemployment rates and education are reported in the census data (Francis et al., 2013). The ABS website allows free access to a number of useful resources, including a community profile option (ABS, 2013c). Further information on local community populations and the resources available are accessible through local government and tourist information websites and in hard-copy publications that they produce.

The information generated from this process can inform prospective planning. For example, if data reveal the community has an ageing population, then planning activities to promote healthy ageing would be strategic. For instance, lobbying local government and investing in training of nursing staff to equip them with the knowledge and skills to deliver appropriate care to this group would be a suitable activity for healthcare services to undertake. These data are useful for nurses to plan and develop projects in rural communities. Table 3.1 provides a useful template for developing a demographic profile.

TABLE 3.1 *Demographic profile.*

VARIABLE	NUMBER	%
Age		
Gender		
Ethnicity		
Marital status		
Household income		
Education level		
Occupation		
Housing		
Language		

Resource base

To effect efficient community programs, detailed knowledge of community resources is warranted. The resource base of any community is guided by the particular strengths of that community, both fiscal and human. If the total population of a community is small, then it follows that the fiscal resource base will be limited. Added to that, if a significant number of people existing in this community are below the poverty line, then the fiscal resource base will be severely limited. On the other hand, a population that is larger and varied in age and socioeconomic status would have a stronger fiscal resource base.

Human resources are not that easy to predict. Human resource bases are constructed by considering the education attainment of the population, the age profile, the social status and the gender mix of that population. For example, a population that is largely made up of single young men (as in some mining communities) will have little interest in investing or engaging with that community's projects (Carrington, Hogg, McIntosh & Scott, 2012). However, the economic base of such a community would be booming, as the buying power would be strong. Alternatively, a community with a large proportion of retirees may have greater capacity and interest to contribute to community life, although the economic base may be less robust. Communities that have high employment opportunities are more likely to experience population and economic growth than those that have diminishing employment. Linked to employment opportunities is the prospect of increased education, health, retail, transport and other services.

Community assets

Most large towns in Australia have begun with an incentive for existing. Consider Wagga Wagga in New South Wales: this community is located on major transport links (air, train and road) between Adelaide, Sydney and Melbourne. The main industries are farming, education, health, retail and tourism. A small number of commercial enterprises exist to support the main industries. These activities afford local employment opportunities that both grow and sustain the community. The city had realised growth in new homes, commercial and industrial properties (Wagga Wagga City Council, 2010). Planning the growth of communities in Australia is the responsibility of local councils. Longitudinal plans that provide the blueprint for decisions that will realise the growth of the community are formulated as is described in the Wagga Wagga plan (see following web link).

http://www.wagga.nsw.gov.au/__data/assets/pdf_file/0016/2914/GROW_WaggaWagga.pdf

Population growth demands attention to service development in key areas, namely education and health. Using Wagga Wagga again as an exemplar: the city has nine pre-schools, 18 government and non-government primary schools, eight government and non-government high schools, a regional TAFE institution and one university. In addition, it showcases Gallery 43 (art space), a school for seniors, a community college for employment and training, and a centre for training (Wagga Wagga City Council, 2012).

Communication networks

Communicating across rural networks presents many challenges. Before the days of electronic systems, communication was slow and its efficiencies questionable. As discussed previously, rural health networks are often intricate as they comprise several health disciplines often complicated by the tyranny of distance between them. Nevertheless, with the advent of high-speed broadband, electronic systems should facilitate an ambience of faultless communication across all sectors. The implementation of a national broadband network that is promoted as the next-generational network will make sure all Australian households and businesses have access to a high-speed system that ensures equitable access to information as well as an efficient communication system (Australian Government, 2013). Once in place, this system should revolutionise health care in rural and remote regions of Australia. Telehealth, e-health, m-health and/or telemedicine, case conferencing, and access to educational and professional development programs offered online will be enhanced, as will the capacity to access information related to individual patients; all these should result in improved health outcomes (Krumm & Ferrari, 2008; McCarthy, 2010; Moffatt & Eley, 2010). The use of telecommunication systems to enhance rural nursing and midwifery health practice is also highlighted in Chapter 2.

Case management and case conferencing

The organisation of health care within the community places the client as the centrepiece of all communication. Case management is one method for ensuring that clients'/patients' care is facilitated. A case manager usually calls the group together, facilitates the communication and coordinates activities of care (Anjou, Boudville & Taylor, 2013; Chouinard et al., 2013; Corvol et al., 2013). This person can emanate from any of the health disciplines: nursing, physiotherapy, social work, for example. Case conferencing is a formal structured process that should occur at regular intervals. Case conferencing brings together all the medical, nursing and allied health personnel involved in the care of the patient. Eliciting the views of all health professionals helps build a total picture of care and results in a holistic approach to patient care. Recording meeting minutes is recommended, as is the generation of an associated action sheet that documents activities to be undertaken, the person/s responsible and the specified time frame (NYS Department of Health, 2013). The case manager is central to helping the client/patient navigate the healthcare system, thus ensuring optimal health outcomes.

Nature and profile of burden of disease

The World Health Organization (WHO) measures the global burden of disease using the disability-adjusted life year (DALY). The DALY is a time-based measure that calculates '... years of life lost due to premature mortality and years of life lost due to time lived in states of less than full health' (WHO, 2013a, para 1). The data obtained from calculating the burden of disease and risk factors inform health planning (Allotey, Reidpath, Kouamé & Cummins, 2003). The WHO website hosts the *Global Health Observatory* from which international health data, analysis of the data, trends and determinants of health can be accessed. The WHO asserts that all nations need to generate accurate health data to inform planning, resource allocations and accountabilities (2013b).

Australia has a world-class healthcare system ranked 32 out of 191 by the WHO (2000). Despite this ranking, Australia, like most western nations, has a growing burden of disease that is exacerbated by increased longevity of the population. The Australian Institute of Health and Welfare (AIHW) reported in 2012 that life expectancy was 79.5 years for men and 84.0 years for women. Aboriginal and Torres Strait Islander Australians, however, can expect to live 12 years less than non-Indigenous Australians (AIHW, 2012). Moreover, Australians (Indigenous and non-Indigenous) who live in rural and remote regions have poorer health compared to those who reside in metropolitan locations (see Chapter 1). Health status is impacted by determinants of health, including social and economic conditions such as education, occupation and wealth, lifestyle, social status, as well as genetic, biological and environmental factors (AIHW, 2012). Understanding the factors that influence health status enables governments to intervene and reduce and/or eradicate the burden created by disease; this then improves individuals' quality of life and the nation's productivity, and it reduces healthcare expenditure.

The AIHW (2012) reports on the burden of disease using the DALY methodology. The data they generate identify the extent and distribution of health problems and quantify key health risks. Cancer is the major disease group causing the greatest disease burden in Australia. This is followed by cardiovascular disease, nervous system and mental health disorders, and chronic respiratory diseases, diabetes and injuries (AIHW, 2012). Risk factors that have been identified as increasing the likelihood of individuals developing these diseases include tobacco smoking, hypertension and obesity, high blood cholesterol and inactivity.

Australian governments (at both state and federal levels) invest in strategies that include research to learn more about causation and treatment of diseases, health interventions, and increasing the population's health literacy to reduce the burden of diseases. Campaigns such as 'It's time to be a swapper', 'World Diabetes Day', 'Walk to Healthy Heart on World Heart Day' and 'Quit Smoking' are designed to raise awareness of risk factors and simple methods that can be adopted to reduce risk. These initiatives, coupled with improving other known risk factors such as socioeconomic status and living conditions, and access to education and health services, are key initiatives advocated and supported by the Australian Government to improve health status for all.

Access and health outcomes

The concentration of the Australian population in metropolitan centres has led to an inequitable distribution of health and other goods and services (See Chapters 1 and 2). Rural and remote locations characteristically have reduced diversity of locally available services compared with metropolitan areas. Access to health and other services, including education and employment, is recognised as a key factor impacting on health outcomes for individuals, groups and populations (AIHW, 2008). As has been highlighted in previous chapters, living in rural and remote areas is inversely correlated with poorer health outcomes compared with people who live in metropolitan areas (AIHW, 2013b; Lee, Nguyen, Hoang & Terry, 2012).

The AIHW (2013b) cautions, however, that access is not the only predictor of poorer health. Environmental issues such as workplaces and risks associated with driving (including speed, long distances and animals on the roads), coupled with higher smoking and alcohol consumption than for metropolitan populations, all adversely impact on the health status of rural and remote communities. Moreover, the higher proportions of Aboriginal and Torres Strait Islander people in rural and remote areas elevate morbidity and mortality data (AIHW, 2013a) compared with metropolitan population data. Aboriginal and Torres Strait Islander people's life expectancy, according to the AIHW, is lower than that of non-Indigenous Australians: Aboriginal and Torres Strait Islander men's life expectancy at birth is 67.2 years, which is 11.5 years less than for non-Indigenous men, and Aboriginal and Torres Strait Islander women's life expectancy at birth is 72.9 years, some 9.7 years less than for non-Indigenous women (AIHW, 2013a). These data indicate that the life expectancy of Aboriginal and Torres Strait Islander people has improved slightly since the 2012 data mentioned previously.

Humphreys and Wakerman (n.d.) argue that the models of health care utilised predominantly in rural and remote settings replicate those used in large metropolitan settings, which, they contend, is not appropriate. Funding of health services is generally related to population density, which clearly disadvantages rural and remote services, although some adjustments to funding are made to accommodate this perversity. Increasing access to healthcare services is being achieved through the use of technology, as discussed earlier in this chapter, and by the adoption of innovative models of care such as the Royal Flying Doctor Service, the Medical Specialist Outreach Program, Rural Women's General Practice Service and primary healthcare services (including general practices and nurse-led services) (Healthinsite, 2013; Humphreys & Wakerman, n.d.).

As discussed in Chapter 2, nurses form the largest group of health professionals and are the most evenly distributed in Australia. As such, nurses are key to improving health outcomes for rural and remote populations. Knowing the community, advocating on their behalf and adopting innovative approaches to practice to best meet the community's needs are vital skills to ensure that practice reflects the principles of cultural responsiveness.

While there has been recognition by all governments of Australia that rural populations are disadvantaged, there is much to be done. Models of care need to be continually evaluated and modified to ensure that rural and remote communities, their families and individuals have access to appropriate health care. Nurses must lead in this endeavour.

Maryanne has accepted a position as the health services manager of a Multiple Purpose Service (MPS) in rural Victoria. Maryanne was told at interview that the services offered by the MPS need to be reviewed and possibly changed and that she would need to engage with the community as part of the process. The MPS is inclusive of acute care, aged care, emergency, respite, mental health and community nursing services. The MPS is located 425 kilometres north east of Melbourne and services a population of approximately 2000 people. Maryanne is not familiar with the community and has never worked in a small service of this type before. She understands that there are no resident medical officers; rather, three general practitioners (GPs) support the MPS. Two of these GPs own and work in the same medical practice. The third GP is employed by an Aboriginal Medical Service that also employs two practice nurses (RN and EN Medication Endorsed) and a nurse practitioner. The nurse practitioner and a number of nursing staff from the MPS have contacted Maryanne congratulating her and indicating that they are looking forward to working with her.

VIGNETTE

Questions

1 What information does Maryanne need to gather before commencing in her new position?
2 What advice would you give Maryanne about collecting data to inform her understanding?
3 Getting to know the community and asking them for their input is an important aspect of Maryanne's work. Suggest methods that Maryanne could use to meet the community and involve them in an ongoing dialogue about the MPS.
4 How should Maryanne engage with MPS staff and external service providers?
5 Maryanne needs to develop a strategic plan that charts the way forward for the MPS. Suggest methods that could be used to achieve this goal.

Summary

Working in rural and remote settings requires knowledge that can be gained by knowing the community. This chapter has highlighted methods to gain understanding that can inform practice and ultimately improve health outcomes.

In this chapter, we have covered:

- the composition of community profiles that comprise features such as the demographics, resources and assets that make up a community
- profile demographics such as age, ethnicity, gender, employment status, income and education level that provide a picture of the population that makes up a community
- community assets, human and fiscal resources, knowledge of the population demographics as elements to be considered when prospectively planning for a community
- the burden of disease impacting on rural communities and factors that influence health status
- communication across rural communities and the recent technological advances that have facilitated greater access to services such as telemedicine, case conferencing and professional development programs for health professionals.

Reflective questions

1 Consider a rural population with which you are familiar. Compile a list of what you know about the features of this community.
2 What are the gaps in the profile you have produced of this community? Where might you obtain any outstanding information?
3 For the community that you have identified, what is the burden of disease? How does this relate to the characteristics of the community that you have identified?
4 What limitations does this community face in respect of equity of access to health and other services?
5 Discuss the role of nurses and midwives in addressing the burden of disease.

References

Allotey, P., Reidpath, D., Kouamé, A. & Cummins, R. (2003). The DALY, context and the determinants of the severity of disease: An exploratory comparison of paraplegia in Australia and Cameroon. *Social Science & Medicine*, 57(5), 949. doi: 10.1016/S0277–9536(02)00463-X

Anjou, M. D., Boudville, A. I. & Taylor, H. R. (2013). Local co-ordination and case management can enhance Indigenous eye care – a qualitative study. *BMC Health Services Research*, 13(1), 255–64. doi: 10.1186/1472–6963–13–255

Australian Bureau of Statistics (ABS). (2013a). 3235.0 – *Population by age and sex, regions of Australia, 2011*. Retrieved May 6, 2013, from http://www.abs.gov.au/ausstats/abs@.nsf/Products/3235.0~2011~Main+Features~Main+Features?OpenDocument

——. (2013b). *Community profiles*. Retrieved September 8, 2013, from http://www.abs.gov.au/websitedbs/censushome.nsf/home/communityprofiles

——. (2013c). *Data & analysis*. Retrieved June 21, 2013, from http://www.abs.gov.au/websitedbs/censushome.nsf/home/data?opendocument – from-banner=LN

Australian Government. (2013). National broadband network. Retrieved September 11, 2013, from http://www.dbcde.gov.au/broadband/national_broadband_network – overview

Australian Institute of Health and Welfare (AIHW). (2008). *Rural, regional and remote health: Indicators of health status and determinants of health*. Rural health series no. 9. Cat. no. PHE 97. Canberra: AIHW.

——. (2012). *Australia's health 2012*. Australia's health series no. 13. Cat. no. AUS 156. Canberra: AIHW.

——. (2013a). Indigenous observatory [Factsheet]. Retrieved November 11, 2013, from http://www.aihw.gov.au/WorkArea/DownloadAsset.aspx?id=10737419014&libID=10737419013

——. (2013b). *Impact of rurality on health status*. Retrieved November 11, 2013, from http://www.aihw.gov.au/rural-health-impact-of-rurality/

Carrington, K., Hogg, R., McIntosh, A. & Scott, J. (2012). Crime talk, FIFO workers and cultural conflict on the mining boom frontier. *Australian Humanities Review*, 53 (Online). Retrieved March 22, 2014, from http://www.australianhumanitiesreview.org/archive/Issue-November-2012/carrington_etal.html

Chouinard, M.-C., Hudon, C., Dubois, M.-F., Roberge, P., Loignon, C., Tchouaket, É., … Sasseville, M. (2013). Case management and self-management support for frequent users with chronic disease in primary care: A pragmatic randomized controlled trial. *BMC Health Services Research*, 13(1), 1–13. doi: 10.1186/1472–6963–13–49

Community profiling. (2004). Retrieved September 8, 2013, from http://www.barnardos.org.uk/communityprofiling.pdf

Corvol, A., Moutel, G., Gagnon, D., Nugue, M., Saint-Jean, O. & Somme, D. (2013). Ethical issues in the introduction of case management for elderly people. *Nursing Ethics*, 20(1), 83–95. doi: 10.1177/0969733012452685

Francis, K., Chapman, Y., Hoare, K. & Birks, M. (2013). *Australia and New Zealand Community as partner: Theory and practice in nursing* (2nd ed.). Sydney: Wolters Kluwer/Lippincott, Williams & Wilkins.

Healthinsite. (2013). Rural and remote health. Retrieved November 11, 2013, from http://www.healthinsite.gov.au/topic/rural-and-remote-health

Humphreys, J. & Wakerman, J. (n.d.). Primary health care in rural and remote Australia: Achieving equity of access and outcomes through national reform. Alice Springs: Monash University and Centre for Remote Health Flinders University and Charles Darwin University. Retrieved March 22, 2014, from http://www.health.gov.au/internet/nhhrc/publishing.nsf/Content/16F7A93D8F578DB4C A2574D7001830E9/$File/Primary%20health%20care%20in%20rural%20and%20 remote%20Australia%20-%20achieving%20equity%20of%20access%20and%20 outcomes%20through%20national%20reform%20(J%20Humph.pdf

Krumm, M. & Ferrari, D. V. (2008). Contemporary telehealth and telemedicine applications in audiology. *Audiology Today*, 20(5), 36–41.

Lee, Q., Nguyen, H. B., Auckland, S., Hoang, H. & Terry, D. (2012). Access to health care services in an Australian rural area – a qualitative case study. *International Journal of Annotative Interdisciplinary Research*, 3, 29–36.

McCarthy, M. (2010). Telehealth or tele-education? Providing intensive, ongoing therapy to remote communities. *Studies in Health Technology & Informatics*, 161, 104–11.

Moffatt, J. J. & Eley, D. S. (2010). The reported benefits of telehealth for rural Australians. *Australian Health Review*, 34(3), 276–81. doi: 10.1071/AH09794

New Forest District Council. (2013). Toolkit Guide Three: The community profile questions. Retrieved September 8, 2013, from http://www.newforest.gov.uk/ media/adobe/6/6/TK_three.pdf

New York State Department of Health. (2013). Case coordination and case conferencing. Retrieved October 1, 2013, from http://www.health.ny.gov/ diseases/aids/standards/casemanagement/case_coordination_conferencing.htm

Wagga Wagga City Council. (2010). Grow – Wagga Wagga: A blueprint for continued economic growth of the city 2008 through to 2018. Retrieved November 28, 2013, from http://www.wagga.nsw.gov.au/__data/assets/pdf_file/0016/2914/GROW_ WaggaWagga.pdf

——. (2012). Further education. Retrieved November 28, 2013, from www.waggawaggaaustralia.com.au/schools-and-education/further-education

World Health Organization (WHO). (2000). *World Health Report 2000: Health systems: Improving performance*. Geneva: WHO. Retrieved November 28, 2013, from http://www.who.int/whr/2000/en/whr00_en.pdf

——. (2013a). Global burden of disease. Retrieved October 11, 2013, from http://www.who.int/topics/global_burden_of_disease/en/

——. (2013b). The Global Health Observatory. Retrieved October 11, 2013, from http://www.who.int/healthinfo/en/index.html

The practice of rural nursing and midwifery

4

Jenny Davis, Moira Williamson and Ysanne Chapman

Learning objectives

On completion of this chapter, the reader will be able to:

- describe the rural health workforce

- discuss the role of a rural registered nurse or midwife

- explain the challenges of practising as a registered nurse or midwife in a rural context

- identify methods for ensuring currency of practice

- explain cultural responsiveness and how this concept can be embedded in practice.

Key words

- Rural nursing and midwifery, practice, workforce, education, recency of practice

Chapter overview

This chapter focuses on rural nursing and midwifery practice. For the purposes of discussion, the context of rural practice will include remote area nursing practice encompassing a wide range of health services and settings, including small inpatient and multipurpose facilities, aged care, general practice and community health, outreach services, sole practitioner sites and locally controlled Aboriginal community health services (Francis & Mills, 2011). Nurses and midwives employed in rural and remote health services face numerous challenges that will be discussed.

Introduction

Australia, as highlighted in Chapter 1, is characterised as a large continent in which the majority of the population reside along the coastal perimeters and within urban or regional locations, with over two-thirds living in major cities

(Baxter, Gray & Hayes, 2011). The population in rural and remote areas of Australia is small in comparison to the urban and regional areas of the continent (Baxter et al., 2011). Therefore, as the population dwindles in size, so do the resources available to these rural and remote populations. This affects the ability of an individual to receive the same health care as their urban counterparts (Carey, Wakerman, Humphreys, Buykx & Lindeman, 2013). The provision of healthcare professionals is another issue; it is often difficult to attract and maintain the services of healthcare providers in rural and remote areas of Australia (Yates, Kelly, Lindsay & Usher, 2013).

Nursing and midwifery workforce

Nurses and midwives are the largest group of healthcare professionals within the Australian health workforce (Francis & Mills, 2011). The total number of nurses and midwives registered in 2011 was 326 669; of this number, 283 577 were employed as registered nurses and midwives (Australian Institute of Health and Welfare [AIHW], 2012). Of these, 283 577 midwives accounted for 36 074, and 15 523 reported midwifery as their principal area of practice (AIHW, 2012). To be employed as a registered nurse or midwife in Australia requires the individual to be registered with the Australian Health Practitioner Regulation Agency (AHPRA). This requires the individual to have completed an approved program and educational requirements as determined by the Australian Nursing and Midwifery Accreditation Council.

Initial education of registered nurses and midwives

Nursing education is conducted in the tertiary sector, and individuals can complete either a three-year Bachelor of Nursing program or a four-year double degree, such as a Bachelor of Nursing/Bachelor of Midwifery program. Midwifery education is also undertaken in the tertiary sector; individuals can undertake a three-year Bachelor of Midwifery program or a double degree such as the Bachelor of Nursing/Bachelor of Midwifery. Registered nurses wishing to register as a midwife can choose to undertake a Bachelor of Midwifery or a postgraduate degree in midwifery depending on course availability, preference and/or geographical location.

The average age of the nursing and midwifery workforce in Australia was 44.5 years in 2011, with 38.6% of employed nurses or midwives over 50 years of age (AIHW, 2012). Nursing and midwifery education transferred from a hospital-based apprentice system to education in the tertiary sector in a staged national process from the mid 1980s (Heath, 2002). This means that some registered nurses or midwives who are over 44.5 years of age may not have undertaken any tertiary education. AHPRA requires that all nurses and midwives apply for registration annually. Individuals have to state that they are maintaining the educational requirements, known as 'continuing professional development', that have been sanctioned by the Nursing and Midwifery Board of Australia (2010).

The role of nurses and midwives

Nurses and midwives are vital to sustaining healthcare services in rural and remote locations within Australia (Francis & Mills, 2011). It is well documented that the health of rural and remote communities often lags behind urban and regional communities. Rural health services do not offer the range of specialised health services that are available in urban and regional areas of Australia (Francis & Mills, 2011). This therefore means that healthcare professionals, such as nurses and midwives, need to be multiskilled in their practice and are required to cover a diverse client base with a broad range of healthcare needs (Hegney, 1996; Mills, Birks & Hegney, 2010).

Workforce pressures and recognition of the value of health practitioner role diversity have contributed to multiskilling being considered an effective and continuing workforce strategy (Buykx et al., 2012; Fahey & Monaghan, 2005). As highlighted in Chapter 2, rural nurses' practice is lifespan inclusive, requiring a depth and breadth of knowledge and skills that ensure appropriate health care is provided irrespective of the age of clients. This broad range of skills has been described as 'jack of all trades and master of many' (Hegney, as cited in Mills et al., 2010, p. 33). As the major providers of health care in these contexts, rural nurses and midwives provide holistic care that is inclusive of psychosocial, spiritual and physical care.

Rural and remote health services rely heavily on the nursing and midwifery workforce, and there is a growing argument in favour of the creation of alternative models of care that enable rural and remote practitioners to work to their full scope of practice (Sullivan, Hegney & Francis, 2012). An investigation into the economic value and potential of nurse practitioner models in Australia (Centre for International Economics, 2013) found these models to be increasingly important across a wide range of care settings, providing quality care that is complementary to existing health services, is able to fill clinical service gaps and is more responsive to community needs.

Diverse role requirements in some healthcare settings can create additional challenges for rural and remote nurses and midwives, who are required to work and maintain critical knowledge and practice competency in areas broadly including paediatrics, gerontology, general medical/surgical and mental health. Organisational support for continuing professional development activities for nurses and midwives in rural and remote settings is therefore critical not just for an individual's care, but it is also increasingly recognised as a future investment in workforce supply, creating sustainable health services and playing a vital role in improving the health of rural and remote communities (Buykx et al., 2012; Fahey & Monaghan, 2005; Kidd, Kenny & Meehan-Andrews, 2012).

Rural and remote nurses can therefore be considered different from metropolitan nurses in terms of demographic characteristics, practice context and the diversity of skills required to care for individuals with unique and complex health profiles (Pront, Kelton, Munt & Hutton, 2013). In some contexts, these nurses may also practise with or without support from other health professionals, including medical and allied health personnel (Francis, Bowman & Redgrave, 2002), and ancillary staff such as porters or administrative staff. The literature review by Francis et al. (2002) identifies that registered nurses need to have a wide range of skills in order to provide appropriate health care to rural and remote Australian communities, including interpersonal skills, management ability, knowledge of legal and ethical concepts, advanced clinical practice, education and research.

Despite rural and remote settings often being portrayed negatively in terms of health status and outcomes and access to services, there is increasing evidence of the capacity for nurses and midwives to positively impact on the health of their communities (Pearson, 2008). This is particularly so in areas where there are too few doctors to support existing services. Recommended models that spread clinical workload across more autonomous interdisciplinary teams offer real opportunities for rural nurses and midwives to truly work to their full scope of practice and improve resource efficiency at the point of care (Sullivan et al., 2012). Advanced practice roles for nurses, such as nurse practitioners, and low-risk midwifery-led models for maternity care are clear examples of how rural and remote nurses and midwives are vital not just for the health of these communities, but also for their continuing sustainability (Pearson, 2008). Whilst these models have been found to positively impact on access, efficiency and quality of care across a range of settings, their implementation and acceptance have been embraced in some areas but remain sporadic in others (Centre for International Economics, 2013).

The impact on a rural and remote community of the loss or retention of health professionals can be profound, affecting the availability of health services, as even small changes in population through internal migration or depopulation ultimately flow on to education and other key services in these communities (Bennett, Barlow, Brown & Jones, 2012; Gregory, 2009). There is a growing discussion in relation to the changing demography of rural and remote communities about the impact that population influx or migration can have on nursing and midwifery practice, including the additional pressure placed on health services in regards to the expansion of mining and coal seam gas industries (Hossain et al., 2013). Whilst these issues can pre-empt emotive discussion, there are real and increased concerns for rural and remote communities, particularly in relation to psychosocial impacts of the fly-in, fly-out workforce, changing community structures and overall community mental health (Hossain et al., 2013; Torkington, Larkins & Gupta, 2011; Wakerman, Curry & McEldowney, 2012). For rural and remote Aboriginal and Torres Strait Islander communities, these changing community characteristics and structures may be a reminder of times past when dislocation, dispossession and exclusion were common experiences; these are now slowly being redressed through collaboration and inclusive strategies (Baker, 2010; Torkington et al., 2011).

Rural and remote nurses and midwives often carry increased responsibility, as evidenced by the need for them to be in charge of ward areas, emergency presentations and the health facility simultaneously, coupled with the unpredictable nature of these work environments, limited resources and limited availability of other health professionals and support staff (Gregory, 2009; Hegney, 1996; Kidd et al., 2012; Pront et al., 2013). For rural and remote nurses, there can be additional community responsibility if they are more visible and closely connected to the commonly shared fabric of the community in their personal roles as partner, spouse or parent, for example (Pront et al., 2013). Similarly, other health professionals working in rural and remote communities share the challenges associated with managing highly visible personal and professional relationships amidst raised community expectations (Allan, Ball & Alston, 2008).

In a more positive sense, rural and remote nurses and midwives may achieve or perceive greater professional satisfaction and recognition from role diversity and a more personal level of community engagement and a closer sense of community involvement (Fragar & Depczynski, 2011; Gregory, 2009; Kidd et al., 2012; Yates et al., 2013). A balanced perspective of the positive and negative aspects of work as a rural or remote health practitioner is offered here to exemplify the main challenges of working in rural and remote communities (Bourke, Humphreys, Wakerman & Taylor, 2012).

- Positive aspects – diversity of roles, autonomy, opportunity for innovation, local community connection, witnessing impact of care provided, team-based collaboration in individual patient care.
- Negative aspects – lack of financial and human and structural resources, ageing local workforce, difficulty recruiting new staff, isolation from specialist services and professional development (Bourke et al., 2012, p. 496).

Being both a nurse and a midwife

The context of practice necessarily influences the role of nurses and midwives working in rural settings (Mills et al., 2010). Rural nurses are commonly described as generalist specialists, with practice context influencing the often diverse and multifaceted nature of their roles and responsibilities (Hegney, 1996; Kenny & Duckett, 2003; Pront et al., 2013). The most important influences on these roles have been identified as distance from tertiary facilities, availability of other healthcare professionals, working conditions, and the characteristics of the community in which they work (Kruske et al., 2008).

For midwives working in rural and remote settings, there is often the expectation that they be able to work as both a nurse and a midwife, influenced by both context and prevailing workforce needs (Mills et al., 2010). With the decline in maternity services, there is an associated risk that midwives working in some rural and remote locations may not routinely work with pregnant women, and the practice of transferring women to give birth in larger centres increases the likelihood that confidence and skill levels will decline accordingly (Yates, Usher & Kelly, 2011). Decreasing interest displayed by midwives for work in rural and remote areas may be a consequence of reduced opportunities to work in this area, and this may place the implementation of continuity of care models at further risk (Stewart, Lock, Bentley & Carson, 2012). For rural and remote nurses and midwives, the key to maintaining competence and skills – and thereby confidence – is continued exposure to their areas of practice, challenged further by the need to be cognisant and prepared for the potential unpredictable events and conditions that may present.

Implications of changes to rural health and maternity services

The closure or reconfiguration of some health services, particularly maternity services, over recent years has changed the context in which rural and remote nurses and midwives now practise (Kildea, Kruske & Bowell, 2006). It has been identified that in Australia over the past two decades, more than 50% of small rural maternity units have been closed because of cost, safety and quality concerns amongst workforce pressures (Hoang, Le & Kilpatrick, 2012). Whilst safety considerations are important, these changes effectively shift the costs and risk to rural and remote women, their families and communities (Hoang, Le & Terry, 2014). Increasingly, women are faced with diminished choice and access to maternity services, often having to travel long distances to give birth (Francis et al., 2012).

National and state government reviews of maternity services in Australia have highlighted the inequity in maternity services for rural and remote women; the recommendations from these reviews consistently call for the expansion of primary healthcare models of maternity service delivery (Department of Health and Ageing, 2008; Hirst, 2005; Northern Territory Government, 2007; Western Australia Government, 2007). Indeed, the National Plan (for midwifery) and others increasingly advocate for 'increased access for Australian women to local maternity care by expanding the range of models of care' (Australian Health Ministers' Conference, 2011).

These models of care promote low-risk continuity of care as well as carer, shared care and collaborative arrangements between maternity care providers, with research findings demonstrating these to be safe and acceptable to women (Hatem, Sandall, Devene, Soltani & Gates, 2008; McLachlan et al., 2012). Most importantly, these primary care-based models enable more women to give birth in their community and rural and remote midwives to work within their full scope of practice (Sandall, Soltani, Gates, Shennan & Devane, 2013). However, to date, impediments to the implementation of such new and innovative models of care have been identified to include a lack of funding, new registration requirements, and revisiting the logistics of inter-professional collaborative arrangements, some of which are embedded in traditional models of maternity care (Brown & Dietsch, 2013; Francis et al., 2012; Quinn, Noble, Seale & Ward, 2013).

Social determinants of health and nursing and midwifery practice

In addition to the skills identified by Francis et al. (2002), nurses and midwives employed in rural and remote areas of Australia need to have an understanding of the social determinants that affect their local communities (Mills et al., 2010). It is well documented that individuals living in rural and remote areas of Australia are more likely to experience poorer health status and outcomes (Kidd et al., 2012) and are disadvantaged due to geographical isolation and limited availability of resources for education, health and transport (Russell et al., 2013). There is higher unemployment and other social issues that affect their health and wellbeing (Mills et al., 2010).

Australia is well known for its extreme weather events, and the impact of prolonged or severe weather events such as drought, floods and bushfires can profoundly impact on the health and wellbeing of rural and remote communities, both short and long term. These events, together with the more recent economic downturn, have contributed to a further decline in other services, not just health services, in some regions of Australia (Bennett et al., 2012).

The synergy that exists between rural and remote communities and their social and physical environments means that environmental influences such as drought consequentially impact on individual and community health. This relationship has been highlighted in studies examining the impact of prolonged drought and other events on the health of rural and remote communities, with increased risk of depression and/or suicide (Kõlves, Kõlves & De Leo, 2013).

Cultural responsiveness

Cultural responsiveness is an inclusive concept that informs situational interaction with culturally diverse populations, groups and individuals (Gill & Babacan, 2012) and comprises cultural competence and cultural safety. Cultural competence '… implies understanding and sensitivity of different cultural beliefs and practices' (Francis & Chapman, 2011, p. 239), while cultural safety refers to being safe for people and not being exposed to physical or emotional harm and not being denied self-identity by respecting others (Gill & Babacan, 2012).

Nurses and midwives need to understand the concept of cultural safety and demonstrate respect for diversity and difference across society, and to incorporate these principles into their everyday practice. By understanding the concept and principles of cultural safety, nurses and midwives have the potential to ensure that the individual, group or community is involved in their care, making informed choices and receiving care that suits their particular needs (Williamson & Harrison, 2010).

To fully appreciate the concept of cultural safety, nurses and midwives are required to understand how history and power relationships have affected the health of Aboriginal and Torres Strait Islander individuals (Spence 2003; Kruske, Kildea & Barclay, 2006). Nurses and midwives need to reflect on how the culture of the healthcare institution or healthcare provision impacts on the individual receiving care (Spence, 2003). The aim of cultural safety is to allow the healthcare needs to be 'determined' by the individual (Spence, 2003). Not all Australian nurses and midwives understand the meaning of cultural safety as there has been little education on Aboriginal and Torres Strait Islander health issues in the past (Williamson & Harrison, 2010).

The Australian Nursing and Midwifery Council (ANMC, 2007) recommended that a discrete course/subject on Aboriginal and Torres Strait Islander health, history and culture be included in all nursing and midwifery programs leading to registration (Williamson & Harrison, 2010). The ANMC National Competency Standards for the Registered Nurse (2007) also state that registered nurses need to practise 'in a way that acknowledges the dignity, culture, values, beliefs and rights of individuals/groups'. The National Competency Standards for the Midwife state that midwives need to ensure 'that midwifery practice is culturally safe' (ANMC, 2010).

Johnstone and Kanitsaki (2007) undertook a study to explore healthcare professionals' understanding of the concept of cultural safety. This study explored how the concept of cultural safety was adapted when health professionals were providing care for culturally diverse populations, which was not the original intent of the concept of 'cultural safety' (Williamson & Harrison, 2010). The findings of this study indicated that health professionals did not fully comprehend the meaning of cultural safety (Johnstone & Kanitsaki, 2007). Participants within the study recognised the importance of communicating effectively and providing 'safe care'. However, they did not take into account the social determinants that may have impacted on an individual's wellbeing (Williamson & Harrison, 2010).

Being a culturally responsive nurse or midwife is not limited to interaction with Aboriginal and Torres Strait Islander Australians. As Australia is a multicultural society, nurses and midwives must accommodate and be responsive to the needs of all people, including minority groups such as refugees. In 2010–2011, a total of 13 799 refugee visas were granted by the Australian Government. Some of these refugees settled in rural areas of Australia. Their resettlement to rural areas is related to employment opportunities (Colic-Peisker & Tilbury, 2006). However, refugees located in rural areas of Australia experience greater health inequalities, and their need for primary healthcare services is noteworthy (Sypek, Clugston & Phillips, 2008). This, in turn, creates challenges for rural communities to meet their healthcare needs. A whole-of-community approach to address the needs of vulnerable groups – one that is inclusive of refugees and that capitalises on available resources and is consistent with policy at all levels of government – is recommended.

Anonymity and ethical practice

The nature of living in rural communities, the underlying culture and the way people live their lives can be very different to that of people residing in metropolitan areas. There inherently exists both complexity and greater visibility in personal and professional relationships that are unique to living and working in rural communities, with each carrying benefits and risks (Pront et al., 2013; McConnell-Henry, Chapman & Francis, 2010). The greater likelihood that individuals are well known to nurses and midwives working in rural and remote settings can carry with it a greater emotional burden, particularly when outcomes are poor and they are directly involved in care delivery (Fragar & Depczynski, 2011; McConnell-Henry et al., 2010).

Working and living in rural communities present an additional challenge for rural nurses and midwives as previously discussed in Chapter 2: they are simultaneously members of the community and healthcare providers to the community (Mills, Francis & Bonner, 2007; McConnell-Henry et al., 2010). In this way, personal and professional boundaries are both complex and complicated; the closeness and dynamic nature of relationships and expectations of these communities have the potential to bring an additional layer of complexity to the ethics of care, decision-making and privacy in these settings (Allan et al., 2008; Lea & Cruickshank, 2007).

Maintaining recency of practice

Demonstrating currency of practice is a requirement for annual registration for all nurses and midwives (Nursing and Midwifery Board of Australia, 2010). Meeting this licensure requirement is generally achieved through participating in professional development and educational activities that meet the requirements stipulated by the regulatory authority. Rural nurses and midwives have reported difficulties in accessing continuing professional development and education, citing cost and logistics of access and transport, and limited availability of staff for backfill (Kildea et al., 2006).

Various strategies have been suggested to improve access to professional development opportunities for rural and remote nurses and midwives, including distance learning facilitated through internet services and videoconferencing (Ireland et al., 2007). The promise and potential for telecommunication improvements, such as the National Broadband Network to help overcome some of the geographical and cost barriers, are yet to be fully delivered to all rural and remote communities. Nevertheless, the internet (providing the geographical location supports its use) is invaluable in enabling individuals to access continuing professional education resources.

Some health departments in Australia provide ongoing education for registered nurses and midwives. For example, Queensland Health has initiated the Nursing and Midwifery Staff Development Framework, which includes strategies and education for continuing professional development (Queensland Health, 2010). Professional bodies such as the Australian College of Nursing and the Australian College of Midwives also provide online resources and continuing education programs for the benefit of their membership.

It is not only the internet that provides access for registered nurses and midwives to maintain their professional development. Some universities within Australia have satellite campuses or have developed e-learning technology to provide education for nursing and midwifery students in regional, rural and remote areas (Davis et al., 2012; Clark & Piercey, 2012; Lane-Krebs, 2012). In addition to geographical isolation, rural and remote nurses and midwives can be challenged by professional and social isolation, associated security and safety concerns, and limits to intercollegial professional development opportunities (Bennett et al., 2012). These issues can contribute to increased stress and decreased morale and altogether significantly increase the risk of staff attrition (Bennett et al., 2012).

An examination of the Australian remote area nursing workforce previously identified a maldistribution of midwives throughout Australia and a decline in the number of nurses with midwifery and child health qualifications (Lenthall et al., 2011). Contributing factors, particularly those impacting on remote areas, include changing preregistration education programs for midwives and nursing specialties (Lenthall et al., 2011). As a consequence of an ageing nursing and midwifery workforce, some employers have increased support for remote area nurses to undertake midwifery education (Lenthall et al., 2011). Management support for continuing professional development for rural and remote nurses has been identified as critical to workforce retention (Hegney, 1996); this is even more so for new graduates who need to be supported to become this future workforce. Conflicting expectations have been raised where management seek work-ready, highly capable graduates or new staff, yet new graduates and new staff need to be supported in their transition to the challenges of rural and remote settings if they are to remain (Bennett et al., 2012).

These issues, amongst others, will continue to challenge the professions of nursing and midwifery, and education providers and regulatory bodies must remain vigilant to the needs of rural and remote communities and their workforce – because one health practitioner does not necessarily fit all contexts.

Henry is a registered nurse and has a postgraduate midwifery qualification. He currently works in a maternity unit in a large metropolitan public hospital as a midwife. He travels an hour each way to work, and that is impacting on the time he is able to spend with his family.

VIGNETTE

Henry and his wife have a young family consisting of two girls aged four years and two years, and they are expecting their third child. Henry and his wife have decided to relocate to a rural community as they believe that the children will have a better quality of life. Henry has some reservations, however, about being highly visible within the community and about knowing people who he will care for as a nurse and midwife.

Henry has accepted a position at a small hospital in the community to which they will be relocating. The community has a population of 2500 people that is inclusive of a small number of Sudanese refugees and people who identify as Aboriginals and Torres Strait Islanders. The hospital has a small emergency department staffed by nurses and supported by the two local general practitioners, a general medical and surgical ward, and a small maternity unit. The annual birthing rate for the hospital is 30 births. Henry has been told that he will work primarily as a generalist nurse and will be expected to work in all areas and, on occasion, depending on need, will be rostered to the maternity ward.

Questions
1 How should Henry prepare for his new role?
2 What will be the challenges that Henry faces and what advice would you offer?
3 What initiatives should the hospital have in place to support Henry when he commences work?

》

4 List methods that Henry can utilise to ensure that he is able to demonstrate that his practice as both a nurse and midwife is current.
5 Consider the implications of working with and caring for people who you know.

Summary

In this chapter, we have covered:

- the rural health workforce that is inclusive of nurses and midwives
- the initial education of nurses and midwives
- the role of rural nurses and midwives
- the dual role of nurse and midwife
- implications of changes to rural health and maternity services
- social determinants and nursing and midwifery practice
- cultural responsiveness
- anonymity and ethical practice
- maintaining recency of practice.

The roles of nurses and midwives in rural and remote areas of Australia have been discussed. The challenges of working as registered nurses and midwives in these locations were presented. Nurses and midwives need to be resilient and multiskilled. They are required to deal with emergencies without the added resources – such as medical teams – that their urban colleagues can call on. They are also employed in small communities and therefore may know the individual to whom they are providing care. This can cause ethical dilemmas and high expectations from the community members. On the other hand, the closeness of working in a small community can provide greater satisfaction for the nurses and midwives employed in these healthcare settings.

Ongoing professional development is another area that may add to the feeling of isolation. Nurses and midwives rely on the health services to provide ongoing education rather than travel long distances to attend conferences or seminars. Internet technology (IT) is assisting. However, this is dependent on IT service provision being available.

To maintain a nursing and midwifery workforce for rural and remote areas of Australia, new approaches to practice may be required that enable both nurses and midwives to provide 'continuity of care' to the community. This will improve both health outcomes and work satisfaction.

Reflective questions

1 How can nurses and midwives employed in rural and remote areas be supported?
2 How can health services improve nurses' and midwives' satisfaction with their roles?
3 What can nurses and midwives do to ensure that their practice is culturally responsive?
4 Identify ways that rural nurses and midwives can ensure that they are current in their knowledge and practice.
5 Identify methods that rural nurses and midwives can utilise to negotiate caring for someone who they know.

References

Allan, J., Ball, P. & Alston, M. (2008). 'You have to face your mistakes in the street': The contextual keys that shape health service access and health workers' experiences in rural areas. *Rural and Remote Health*, 8(1), 1–10.

Australian Health Ministers' Conference. (2011). *National Maternity Services Plan*. Canberra: Commonwealth of Australia.

Australian Institute of Health and Welfare (AIHW). (2012). *National health workforce*. Series no. 2. Cat. no. HWL 48. Canberra: AIHW.

Australian Nursing and Midwifery Council. (2007). National competency standards for the registered nurse. Retrieved November 28, 2013, from www.nursingmidwiferyboard.gov.au/documents/default.aspx?record=WD10%2F1342&dbid=AP&chksum=N5ws04xdBl...

——. (2010). National competency standards for the midwife. Retrieved November 28, 2013, from www.nursingmidwiferyboard.gov.au/documents/default.aspx?record=WD10%2F1350&dbid=AP&chksum=Yp0233q3xm...

Baker, J. (2010). Fear of flying. *Rural Society*, 20, 21–34.

Baxter, J., Gray, M. & Hayes, A. (2011). Families in regional, rural and remote Australia. [Factsheet]. Melbourne: Australian Institute of Family Studies.

Bennett, P., Barlow, V., Brown, J. & Jones, D. (2012). What do graduate nurses want from jobs in rural/remote Australian communities? *Journal of Nursing Management*, 20, 485–90.

Bourke, L., Humphreys, J. S., Wakerman, J. & Taylor, J. (2012). Understanding rural and remote health: A framework for analysis in Australia. *Health & Place*, 18, 496–503.

Brown, M. & Dietsch, E. (2013). The feasibility of caseload midwifery in rural Australia: A literature review. *Women and Birth*, 26(1), e1–e4. doi: 10.1016/j.wombi.2012.08.003

Buykx, P., Humphrey, J. S., Tham, R., Kinsman, L., Wakerman, J., Asaid, A. & Tuohey, K. (2012). How do small rural primary health care services sustain themselves in a constantly changing health system environment? *BMC Health Services Research*, 12(81).

Carey, T., Wakerman, J., Humphreys, J., Buykx, P. & Lindeman, M. (2013). What primary health care services should residents of rural and remote Australia be able to access? A systematic review of "core" primary health care services. *BMC Health Services Research*, 13(178).

Centre for International Economics. (2013). *Responsive patient-centred care: The economic value and potential of nurse practitioners in Australia*. Final Report prepared for the Australian College of Nurse Practitioners. Canberra: Centre for International Economics. Retrieved November 28, 2013, from http://acnp.org.au/sites/default/files/docs/final_report_value_of_community_nps.pdf

Clark, S. & Piercey, C. (2012). E-learning provides nursing education in remote areas. *Australian Nursing Journal*, 20(4), 49. Retrieved March 24, 2014, from http://web.ebscohost.com/ehost/pdfviewer/pdfviewer?sid=934226e3-a02c-49d4-962d-29c3b0e07b07%40sessionmgr115&vid=2&hid=114

Colic-Peisker, V. & Tilbury, F. (2006). Employment niches for recent refugees: Segmented labour market in twenty-first century Australia. *Journal of Refugee Studies*, 19(2), 203–29. doi: 10.1093/jrs/fej016

Davis, D., Foureur, M., Clements, V., Brodie, P. & Herbison, P. (2012). The self-reported confidence of newly graduated midwives before and after their first year of practice in Sydney, Australia. *Women and Birth*, 25(3), e1–e10. doi: 10.1016/j.wombi.2011.03.005

Department of Health and Ageing. (2008). *Improving maternity services in Australia: A discussion paper from the Australian government*. Canberra: DoHA. Retrieved March 24, 2014, from http://www.health.gov.au/internet/main/publishing.nsf/Content/8913DED8386618A5CA257BF0001B0A26/$File/Improving_Maternity_Services_In_Australia.pdf

Fahey, C. M. & Monaghan, J. S. (2005). Australian rural midwives: Perspectives on continuing professional development. *Rural and Remote Health*, 5(468) (Online).

Fragar, L. J. & Depczynski, J. C. (2011). Beyond 50. Challenges at work for older nurses and allied health workers in rural Australia: A thematic analysis of focus group discussions. *BMC Health Services Research*, 11(42).

Francis, K., Bowman, D. & Redgrave, M. (2002). Knowledge and skills required by rural nurses to meet the challenging work environment in the 21st century: A review of the literature. *National Review of Nursing Education in 2002: Literature Reviews* (pp. 154–215). Canberra: Commonwealth of Australia.

Francis, K. & Chapman, Y. (2011). Cultural competence. In D. Kralik & A. van Loon (Eds.), *Community nursing in Australia* (pp. 235–66). Milton: Wiley.

Francis, K., McLeod, M., McIntyre, M., Mills, J., Miles, M. & Bradley, A. (2012). Australian rural maternity services: Creating a future or putting the last nail in the coffin. *Australian Journal of Rural Health*, 20, 281–4.

Francis, K. & Mills, J. (2011). Sustaining and growing the rural nursing and midwifery workforce: Understanding the issues and isolating directions for the future. *Collegian*, 18, 55–60. doi: 10.1016/j.colegn.2010.08.003

Gill, G. K. & Babacan, H. (2012). Developing a cultural responsiveness framework in healthcare systems: An Australian example. *Diversity & Equality in Health & Care*, 9(1), 45–55. Retrieved March 24, 2014, from http://web.ebscohost.com/ehost/pdfviewer/pdfviewer?sid=a08da8b1–1237–447c-980a-57d4efc349da%40sessionmgr110&vid=2&hid=122

Gregory, G. (2009). Impact of rurality on health practices and services: Summary paper to the inaugural rural and remote health scientific symposium. *Australian Journal of Rural Health*, 17, 49–52.

Hatem, M., Sandall, J., Devene, D., Soltani, H. & Gates, S. (2008). Midwife-led versus other models of care for childbearing women. *Cochrane Database of Systematic Reviews*, 4, CD004667. doi: 10.1002/14651858.CD004667.pub2.

Heath, P. (2002). *National Review of Nursing Education 2002*. Canberra: Commonwealth of Australia.

Hegney, D. (1996). The status of rural nursing in Australia: A review. *Australian Journal of Rural Health*, 4, 1–10.

Hirst, C. (2005). *Re-birthing: Report of the review of maternity services in Queensland*. Brisbane: Queensland Health. Retrieved March 24, 2014, from http://www.qcmb.org.au/media/pdf/Rebirthing%20report.pdf

Hoang, H., Le, Q. & Kilpatrick, S. (2012). Small rural maternity units without caesarian delivery capabilities: Is it safe and sustainable in the eyes of health professionals in Tasmania? *Rural and Remote Health*, 12(3), 1–11.

Hoang, H., Le, Q. & Terry, D. (2014). Women's access needs in maternity care in rural Tasmania, Australia: A mixed methods study. *Women and Birth*, 27(1), 9–14. doi: 10.1016/j.wombi.2013.02.001

Hossain, D., Gorman, D., Chapelle, B., Mann, W., Saal, R. & Penton, G. (2013). Impact of the mining industry on the mental health of landowners and rural communities in southwest Queensland. *Australasian Psychiatry*, 21(1), 32–7.

Ireland, J., Bryers, H., Van Teijlingen, E., Hundley, V., Farmer, J., Harris, F.,... Caldow, J. (2007). Competencies and skills for remote and rural maternity care: A review of the literature. *Journal of Advanced Nursing*, 58(2), 105–15.

Johnstone, M-J. & Kanitsaki, O. (2007). An exploration of the notion and nature of the construct of cultural safety and its applicability to the Australian health care context. *Journal of Transcultural Nursing*, 18(3), 247–56. doi: 10.1177/1043659607301304

Kenny, A. & Duckett, S. (2003). Educating for rural nursing practice. *Journal of Advanced Nursing*, 44(6), 613–22. doi: 10.1046/j.0309–2402.2003.02851.x

Kidd, T., Kenny, A. & Meehan-Andrews, T. (2012). The experience of general nurses in rural Australian emergency departments. *Nurse Education in Practice*, 12, 11–15.

Kildea, S., Kruske, S. & Bowell, L. (2006). Maternity emergency care: Short course in maternity emergencies for remote area staff with no midwifery qualifications. *Australian Journal of Rural Health*, 14, 111–15. doi: 10.1111/j.1440–1584.2006.00785.x

Kõlves, K., Kõlves, K. E. & De Leo, D. (2013). Natural disasters and suicidal behaviours: A systematic literature review. *Journal of Affective Disorders*, 146(1), 1–14. doi: 10.1016/j.jad.2012.07.037

Kruske, S., Kildea, S. & Barclay, L. (2006). Cultural safety and maternity care for Aboriginal and Torres Strait Islander Australians. *Women and Birth*, 19(3), 73–7. doi: 10.1016/j.wombi.2006.07.001

Kruske, S., Lenthall, S., Kildea, S., Knight, S., Mackay, B. & Hegney, D. (2008). Rural and remote area nursing. In D. Brown & H. Edwards (Eds.), *Lewis's medical–surgical nursing: Assessment and management of clinical problems* (pp. 200–15). Marrickville, NSW: Elsevier.

Lane-Krebs, K. (2012). No picket fences. *Australian Nursing Journal*, 20(4), 47 (Online).

Lea, J. & Cruickshank, M. T. (2007). The experience of new graduate nurses in rural practice in New South Wales. *Rural and Remote Health*, 7, 814. Retrieved March 24, 2014, from http://www.rrh.org.au/publishedarticles/article_print_814.pdf

Lenthall, S., Wakerman, J., Opie, T., Dunn, S., MacLeod, M., Dollard, M., ... Knight, S. (2011). Nursing workforce in very remote Australia, characteristics and key issues. *Australian Journal of Rural Health*, 19, 32–7. doi: 10.1111/j.1440–1584.2010.011714.x

McConnell-Henry, T., Chapman, Y. & Francis, K. (2010). Indigenous and remote health: Rural nursing – looking after people we know. *Australian Nurses Journal*, 17(8), 42.

McLachlan, H., Forster, D., Davey, M., Farrell, T., Gold, L., Biro, M., ... Waldenstrom, U. (2012). Effects of continuity of care by a primary midwife (caseload midwifery) on caesarian section rates in women of low obstetric risk: The COSMOS randomised controlled trial. *British Journal of Obstetrics and Gynaecology*, 119(12), 1483–92.

Mills, J., Birks, M. & Hegney, D. (2010). The status of rural nursing in Australia: 12 years on. *Collegian*, 17, 30–7.

Mills, J., Francis, K. & Bonner, A. (2007). Live my work: Rural nurses and their multiple perspectives of self. *Journal of Advanced Nursing*, 59(6), 583–90. doi: 10.1111/j.1365–2648.2007.04350.x

Northern Territory Government. (2007). *Maternity services review in the Northern Territory*. Darwin: NT Government. Retrieved March 24, 2014, from

http://digitallibrary.health.nt.gov.au/prodjspui/bitstream/10137/240/3/
Maternity%20Services%20Review%20-%20December%202007%20.pdf

Nursing and Midwifery Board of Australia. (2010). *Recency of practice registration standard.* Canberra: ANMC.

Pearson, A. (2008). Claims, contradictions and country life in Australia: The evidence on rural nursing and midwifery. *International Journal of Nursing Practice,* 14, 409–10.

Pront, L., Kelton, M., Munt, R. & Hutton, A. (2013). Living and learning in a rural environment: A nursing student perspective. *Nurse Education Today,* 33, 281–5. doi: 10.1016/j.nedt.2012.05.026

Queensland Health. (2010). *Building blocks of lifelong learning: A framework for nurses and midwives in Queensland.* Brisbane: Queensland Government. Retrieved March 24, 2014, from http://www.health.qld.gov.au/nmoq/documents/qhnmsdf.pdf

Quinn, E., Noble, J., Seale, H. & Ward, J. E. (2013). Investigating the potential for evidence-based midwifery-led services in very remote Australia: Viewpoints from local stakeholders. *Women and Birth,* 26(4), 254–9. doi: 10.1016/j.wombi.2013.07.005

Russell, D. J., Humphreys, J., Ward, B., Chisholm, M., Buykx, P., McGrail, M. & Wakerman, J. (2013). Helping policy-makers address rural health access problems. *Australian Journal of Rural Health,* 21(2), 61–71. doi: 10.1111/ajr.12023

Sandall, J., Soltani, H., Gates, S., Shennan, A. & Devane, D. (2013). Midwife-led continuity models versus other models of care for childbearing women (Review). *Cochrane Database of Systematic Reviews,* 8, CD004667. doi: 10.1002/14651858.CD004667.pub3.

Spence, D. (2003). Nursing people from cultures other than one's own: A perspective from New Zealand. *Contemporary Nurse,* 15(3), 222–31. doi: 10.5172/conu.15.3.222

Stewart, L., Lock, R., Bentley, K. & Carson, V. (2012). Meeting the needs of rural and regional families: Educating midwives. *Collegian,* 19(4), 187–8.

Sullivan, E., Hegney, D. & Francis, K. (2012). Victorian rural emergency care – a case for advancing nursing practice. *International Journal of Nursing Practice,* 18, 226–32.

Sypek, S., Clugston, G. & Phillips, C. (2008). Critical health infrastructure for refugee resettlement in rural Australia: Case study of four rural towns. *Australian Journal of Rural Health,* 16(6), 349–54. doi: 10.1111/j.1440–1584.2008.01015.x

Torkington, A. M., Larkins, S. & Gupta, T. S. (2011). The psychosocial impacts of fly-in fly-out and drive-in drive-out mining on mining employees: A qualitative study. *Australian Journal of Rural Health,* 19, 135–41.

Wakerman, J., Curry, R. & McEldowney, R. (2012). Fly in/fly out health services: The panacea or the problem? *Rural and Remote Health,* 12, 2268 (Online). Retrieved March 24, 2014, from http://www.rrh.org.au/articles/subviewaust.asp?ArticleID=2268

Western Australia Government. (2007). *Improving maternity services: Working together across Western Australia. A policy framework*. Perth: WA Department of Health. Retrieved March 24, 2014, from http://www.healthnetworks.health.wa.gov.au/docs/Improving_Maternity_Choices-Summary.pdf

Williamson, M. & Harrison, L. (2010). Providing culturally appropriate care: A literature review. *International Journal of Nursing Studies*, 47(6), 761–9. doi: 10.1016/j.ijnurstu.2009.12.012

Yates, K., Kelly, J., Lindsay, D. & Usher, K. (2013). The experience of rural midwives in dual roles as nurse and midwife: "I'd prefer midwifery but I chose to live here". *Women and Birth*, 26, 60–4.

Yates, K., Usher, K. & Kelly, J. (2011). The dual role of rural midwives: The potential for role conflict and impact on retention. *Collegian*, 18, 107–13. doi: 10.1016/j.colegn.2011.04.002

5 Pregnancy, paternity and parenting in rural communities

Margaret McLeod, Maureen Miles, John Rosenberg and Peta Lea Gale

Learning objectives On completion of this chapter, the reader will be able to:

- identify the unique needs of rural families in accessing health care

- describe normal pregnancy care and recognise the importance of involving fathers in pregnancy and parenting

- discuss child and family health, including immunisation targets

- recognise vulnerable groups and specific care needs

- identify the needs of children exposed to life-limiting illnesses.

Key words Pregnancy care, paternal role, immunisation, life-limiting illness, vulnerable groups

Chapter overview

This chapter provides a snapshot of rural health care from the perspective of young families. It captures pregnancy care models, involvement of fathers in birthing and caring roles, the promotion of health and wellbeing in children, identification of vulnerable groups, and the support of children with life-limiting illnesses.

Introduction

Healthcare access and equity continue to be significant issues for rural Australians, particularly for women and their young families. The centralisation of services to regional, urban and metropolitan areas has led to enforced travel to access health care or, alternatively, reliance on intermittent outreach services to outlying communities. Thus, the health and wellbeing of this rural cohort require special consideration to ensure optimum health outcomes. Health service and professional regulatory authority reforms highlighted in previous chapters pose issues for rural nurses who are also midwives and for those who hold midwifery-only qualifications; these are further discussed in this chapter.

Pregnancy

In 2009, the Chief Nurse and Midwifery Officer, Rosemary Bryant, led a review of maternity services on behalf of the Federal Government. Subsequently, *Improving Maternity Services in Australia: The Report of the Maternity Services Review* was released following extensive consultation (Commonwealth of Australia, 2009). All contributors acknowledged that 'safe, high-quality and accessible cared *based on informed choice* must be the goal' (p. iii), with these factors being central to future policy development and implementation.

Notwithstanding the quality aims above, rural women of child-bearing age continue to have limited birthing choices. This paucity of choice is linked to 'safety and quality considerations and the availability of an appropriate workforce' (Commonwealth of Australia, 2009, p. 1). While there has been a recognised workforce shortfall for doctors, the Commonwealth of Australia (2009) reports that midwives continue to be well distributed across rural Australia. Homer, Brodie and Leap (2008) note that in some rural and remote areas, 'the local midwife is also the local nurse', with numerous challenges arising from this dual role (p. 11) (previously referred to in Chapters 2 and 4). One of the major challenges is maintaining or proving competency of midwifery practice. Consequently, the number of midwives in rural areas is predicted to decrease, given the recent changes in re-licensing standards imposed by the Australian Health Practitioner Regulation Agency (Francis, McLeod, McIntyre, Mills & Bradley, 2012). Unless regulatory authorities, government agencies and healthcare facilities take significant steps to support rural clinicians with double licensure, many will relinquish their midwifery registrations. This lack of suitable staff will further impact on the number of rural women being forced to leave their communities to access routine pregnancy care.

The exodus of women from their rural communities to access care is not new; for some decades maternity services have closed owing to fiscal constraints, centralisation of services and workforce inadequacies. A study by Dietsch, Davies, Shackleton, Alston and McLeod (2008) revealed that enforced travel away from local support networks often leads to family dislocation and financial hardship. While enforced travel is problematic for many rural families, it is particularly problematic for Aboriginal and Torres Strait Islander women, as they must leave country and travel in isolation to distant health facilities to give birth. Eckermann et al. (2006) assert that many Aboriginal and Torres Strait Islander people experience culture shock when they are hospitalised; this is characterised by 'fear, isolation, withdrawal, dependency, depression and powerlessness' (p. 135). All rural healthcare providers who practise and engage with Aboriginal and Torres Strait Islander Australian families should be aware that the NSW Department of Community Services (2009) provides valuable information.

Useful website:

Working with Aboriginal people and communities: A practice resource
http://www.community.nsw.gov.au/docswr/_assets/main/documents/working_with_aboriginal.pdf

Isolation means that ready access to healthcare professionals is scarce. Thus, when rural women want to confirm a suspected pregnancy, they may resort to purchasing a pregnancy kit from their local pharmacy or general store to make a self-diagnosis.

Maternity models of care are based on continuity of care principles and may be difficult to realise in rural areas. These models should provide a mechanism for women to stay, for all or a greater part of their pregnancies, with their partners, families and communities. Predominantly, rural models of care comprise general practitioner-led, shared care midwife/general practitioner, shared care midwife/general practitioner/obstetrician or obstetrician-led. Regardless of who provides the care, a comprehensive assessment should be undertaken during the initial consultation. It should include:

- estimated due date (EDD)
- routine antenatal blood screening
- routine blood pressure screening
- routine urine screening
- palpation – hands-on learning, identification and assessment
- foetal movement
- antenatal education
- exercise in pregnancy
- physiological changes in pregnancy (Pairman, Tracy, Thorogood & Pincombe, 2010, p. 441).

The EDD can be calculated manually (Naegle's Rule) or with an 'estimated date of birth' wheel (Macdonald & Magill-Cuerden, 2011; Purrett, 2004). During the first prenatal assessment, the woman should be informed that a normal gestation period lasts from 37 to 42 completed weeks (Macdonald & Magill-Cuerden, 2011). This should be supported by an established timetable of care, for example: 'four-weekly from booking until 28 weeks' gestation, fortnightly until 36 weeks and weekly until birth' (Pairman et al., 2010, p. 433).

While preferred and available models of care may lead to many rural women remaining in their local communities to give birth, others who live significant distances from regional centres may be forced to travel several hundred kilometres to access birthing facilities and suitably qualified health professionals.

When a woman, her partner and supporting others arrive at a birthing centre, they should be welcomed into an environment that is calm, quiet, private and relaxing (Reid-Searl, Dwyer, Moxham, Lovegrove & Applegarth, 2012). If the woman is an Aboriginal and Torres Strait Islander Australian, an Aboriginal and Torres Strait Islander support worker could be contacted for the purpose of providing or guiding culturally appropriate care.

Factors that impact on the birthing process for all women are the birth passage, the foetus (the passenger), the relationship between the passage and the passenger, physiological forces of labour and psychosocial considerations (Reid-Searl et al., 2012). It is important for rural women and those who support them to be aware of the stages leading up to and following birth. Knowing what to expect can be reassuring.

Women can experience discomfort and/or pain during the birthing process, and ideally preferences for pain management should have been discussed prior to presentation to the birthing facility. Women may arrive with a Birthing or Vision Plan, which they may adhere to or override, in the course of the birthing process. Macdonald and Magill-Cuerden (2011) note that 'understanding and manifestation of pain will be influenced by cultural experiences of both the woman and her caregivers' (p. 523). Therefore, it is important for caregivers to recognise that their attitudes and beliefs may impact on pain experiences and coping mechanisms for women while birthing. Comfort and pain management options during birthing are presented in Table 5.1.

When the baby is safely born, the clinician manages the third stage, which involves administering an oxytocic drug as per facility protocol, clamping and cutting the umbilical cord, and waiting for signs of placental separation. This latter event is signalled by the uterus becoming globular in shape and the fundus rising, followed by a gush or trickle of blood from the vagina, with the

TABLE 5.1 *Pain management options during birthing.*

NON-PHARMACOLOGICAL	PHARMACOLOGICAL
Massage	Analgesics
	Oral/IM/IV narcotics
Aromatherapy	Inhalational analgesia
Music therapy	Regional anaesthesia
Distraction therapy	Epidural block/infusion
Water therapy	Spinal block
Relaxation/breathing techniques	Local anaesthesia
	Pudendal block
	Perineal infiltration
Position changes	
Psychological support	

(Adapted from Reid-Searl et al., 2012, p. 31)

length of the umbilical cord extending (Lowdermilk, Perry, Cashion & Rhodes Alden, 2012).

After birthing, women will have a vaginal discharge (lochia), which may last for six weeks. During the first two to three days it will be red, and then it turns red or brown, which lasts from three to 10 days. Finally, the lochia will become creamy white, with this flow usually lasting 11 to 14 days (Macdonald & Magill-Cuerden, 2011; Reid-Searl et al., 2012).

When the baby is born, it is assessed at one and five minutes, using the Apgar score, which stands for **A**ppearance (colour), **P**ulse (heart rate), **G**rimace (response to stimuli), **A**ctive (tone) and **R**espirations.

While every woman is hoping to have a normal pregnancy and birth, sometimes there are complications. Some are expected, while others come about with no warning. One complication of pregnancy is preterm labour, which occurs between 20 and 37 weeks' gestation. Other obstetrical emergencies include pre-eclampsia, malpresentations such as breech or footling birth, cord prolapse, shoulder dystocia and postpartum haemorrhage. Rural nurses and midwives are encouraged to review their health facility protocols for the emergency management of these situations.

Breastfeeding is encouraged in Australia, and the baby should be fed as soon as possible after the birth. Biologically, breast milk is the best food for infants, and research indicates that the benefits include physiological, nutritional, health, psychological, social, economic and environmental outcomes

(Lutter, 2000; Oddy, 2001; WHO, 2000, as cited in Pairman et al., 2010, p. 636). While breastfeeding is a natural process, some women do not find it to be intuitive. Therefore, clinicians may need to provide information, support, encouragement and assistance to mothers, as well as providing information to partners. Correct attachment is vitally important. Many rural health services employ lactation consultants in regional centres where they provide telephone consultations or outreach services to women in smaller communities.

Useful websites:

Australian Breastfeeding Association
http://www.breastfeeding.asn.au/default.htm

Australian College of Midwives
http://www.midwives.org.au

Australian National Breastfeeding Strategy 2010–2015
http://www.health.gov.au/internet/main/publishing.nsf/Content/aust-breastfeeding-strategy-2010-2015

Finally, many women experience changes in mood following the birth of their baby. 'The mildest and most common form of postpartum mood change is the "baby blues" which occurs in the first few days postpartum and lasts from 24–48 hours' (Pairman et al., 2010, p. 978). During this time women often cry, appear anxious or irritable, and some complain of sleep disturbances. Given that the prevalence of 'baby blues' is approximately 80%, it is regarded as a normal reaction, immediately following childbirth (Pairman et al., 2010). The main intervention is education and support for both mother and father (Elder, Evans & Nizette, 2013). However, for some women the blues can signal the start of clinical depression. The most severe disturbance of mood is puerperal psychosis, which occurs in about 1 in 1000 pregnancies (Elder et al., 2013). Postnatal depression (PND), which sits between the two extremes, affects approximately 15% of child-bearing women, occurring usually within four to six weeks of childbirth (Maternity Centre Association, 2004, as cited in Pairman et al., 2010, p. 978). PND is characterised by 'irritability, anger, low energy levels, and loss of interest and feelings of guilt' (Buist et al., 2008, as cited in Pairman et al., 2010, p. 978). It can last from four to six months but can also last as long as 12 months. Nurses and midwives, using the Edinburgh Depression Scale, can undertake screening. Treatment can include education, counselling and antidepressants (Cox, Holden & Sagovsky, 1987).

Paternity

It is important to involve fathers in antenatal care as it 'enables them to participate in decision-making and be informed about the care pathway and environmental factors that may influence the health of the baby during pregnancy' (Department of Health [DoH], 2012, p. 7). Included in this education are lifestyle factors such as diet, exercise, smoking and drug usage. Education and information about pregnancy and childbirth should be available to women and their partners as well as information pertaining to assessment and intervention, which could include mental health, smoking cessation and immunisation (DoH, 2012). The active involvement of fathers in the care and wellbeing of their unborn children should provide a seamless pathway to participation throughout infancy, childhood and adolescence.

Parenting in rural communities

Child and family health

The specific role and title of maternal and child health nurses differ among the states and territories of Australia. However, these nurses generally provide support for parents and children using a primary healthcare model based in a community healthcare setting. The dual role of this service is to provide basic healthcare assessments for children, from birth to six years of age (this differs from state to state). The major component of this role is related to education of parents/carers, specifically about the normal patterns of growth and development. This role is the first of many in ensuring that children and families are given access to the healthcare information and education that are required to ensure every child is given the opportunity to achieve their full potential in life. One example is the information provided to new parents regarding safe sleeping practices and the relationship to sudden infant death syndrome (SIDS). Up until the mid 1990s, SIDS 'claimed the lives of more infants than any other cause, about 2–4 in 1000' (Barnes & Rowe, 2009, p. 121). Since then, campaigns to inform parents have focused on the following: placing infants on their backs to sleep; keeping bumpers and other loose bedding and soft toys away from sleeping infants; and providing a smoke-free environment (Barnes & Rowe, 2009). Since the introduction of public campaigns, there has been a significant downturn in the death rate, 'with an 84% reduction' (Barnes & Rowe, 2009, p. 121).

Evidence suggests that childhood health and nutrition are major factors in the prevention of chronic diseases in adulthood. It is important to establish healthy eating habits in the preschool age range, as these habits last a lifetime. One of the key determinants of health is maintaining a healthy weight range. However, almost one in four children (23%) are considered obese or overweight (Department of Health and Ageing [DoHA], 2007). Excess weight places significant strain on young bodies, contributing to muscle and bone complaints, cardiovascular disease, some types of cancer, sleep disorders, type 2 diabetes and high blood pressure (DoHA, 2007). Many health problems are preventable by adherence to a healthy lifestyle and good eating habits. Availability and access to good nutritious food, including the five essential food groups (fruit, vegetables, dairy, meat/meat alternatives, and breads and cereals) are essential to aid normal growth and development. Still, many children do not eat the recommended amounts, with some consuming too much sugar or excessive amounts of saturated fat, which is a risk factor for cardiovascular disease (DoHA, 2007).

Useful websites:

Healthy Kids
http://www.healthykids.nsw.gov.au/stats-research.aspx

The Australian *National Child Nutrition and Physical Activity Survey: 2007*
http://www.healthykids.nsw.gov.au/stats-research/national-child-nutrition-and-physical-activity-survey-2007.aspx

Oral/dental care and hygiene are very important in preschool and school-aged children. Good oral hygiene practices are essential in ensuring multiple facets of a child's development. According to Arora et al. (2011), dental caries are one of the most prevalent childhood diseases worldwide. The complications of dental caries can be severe, including severe pain, anxiety, sepsis and sleep loss. Sleep deprivation in children has a significant impact on development, particularly cognitive development, which can cause considerable ongoing learning issues.

According to the Australian Institute of Health and Welfare (AIHW) (2012), children with poor oral health may demonstrate problems in behaviour, peer interaction and school absences, leading to a correlating poor performance at school and lost potential. Poor oral health has proven association with increased risk of chronic disease and mental health issues. Access and equity to dental services have generated enormous debate within the healthcare framework, including the rural context, with particular emphasis on Aboriginal and Torres Strait Islander Australians.

In Australia, current immunisation rates are falling, and greater efforts need to be made to ensure that babies, children and young people are immunised (see Chapter 6). The maternal and child healthcare system plays a vital role in respect to equity of access and early intervention programs.

Useful website:

Immunise Australia Program
http://www.immunise.health.gov.au/

One of the leading causes of injury in preschool children in Australia is injury in and around the home. Common injuries include cuts and abrasions to the face, hands and knees, and green stick and spiral fractures. The two- to five-year age range is most at risk of falls from more than one metre. Among children aged one to 14 years in 2008–2010, the leading causes of death were injuries (34%), cancer (17%) and diseases of the nervous system (11%), with rates of 4.5, 2.2 and 1.5 per 100 000 children, respectively (AIHW, 2012) (see Chapter 6).

There is a range of common complaints that affect babies and children. Respiratory conditions include asthma, bronchitis and pertussis. While asthma remains one of the national health priorities for children, there has been no significant increase in incidence since 2001. Currently, 10% of children in Australia have asthma, the same as for the rest of the population (AIHW, 2012). However, prevalence rates are slightly higher in Aboriginal and Torres Strait Islander children at 14% (AIHW, 2012). Asthma management is featured in Chapter 6.

Dehydration in children is a very real issue, especially in low social economic groups. As Table 5.2 demonstrates, the percentage of water in infants and toddlers is greater, with a larger percentage in the extracellular fluid (ECF). Vomiting and diarrhoea can lead to significant dehydration; this, in turn, will

TABLE 5.2 *Dehydration in infants and toddlers – percentage of water.*

AGE	BODY WEIGHT AS FLUID (%)
Newborn	70–80%, 48% in ECF
Infant in first year	64%, 34% in intracellular fluid (ICF), 30% in ECF
By end of second year	60%, 36% in ICF, 24% in ECF
Puberty	40% in ICF, 20% in ECF

(Adapted from Hazinski, 2013, p. 679)

lead to increased heart rate, which will eventually lead to fatigue, coma and death if not corrected (Glasper & Richardson, 2010).

Finally, it should be noted that Aboriginal and Torres Strait Islander children fare poorly in a number of areas, according to the AIHW (2012), with these children continuing to have higher infant and child death rates than the national rate.

Vulnerable populations

Poor physical, psychological and/or social health represents a significant risk for populations. The epidemiological concept of risk underpins the definition of vulnerability that suggests an individual has the potential to become ill within a given time, with this probability putting the individual at risk of being vulnerable. There are both community and accompanying individual characteristics that are predictive of risk factors, and these include poverty, drug use and living in rural and remote regions (McMurray, 2007).

Risk can be explained in terms of relative and potential risk. Relative risk is described as the risk between groups and their risk of poor health (i.e. those exposed to risk factors and those who are not) (Aday, 1994). With respect to influenza, for example, there is a relative risk of contracting the condition if exposed to someone with the condition; however, there is a relatively low risk if there is no exposure. If additional vulnerabilities are present, such as a low immune system or chronic illness, there is potential that influenza would be contracted. Relative risk, therefore, also reflects the differential vulnerability of divergent groups to poor health. Finally, the concept of risk establishes that everyone is potentially at risk of poor health.

The risk, or potential of risk, might be higher during particular stages of life, for example during the perinatal period. A woman who has had a traumatic birth is at higher risk of poor physical and/or psychological health in the perinatal period because of blood loss, a perineal wound or birthing trauma. These conditions are further exacerbated if there are underlying mental health disorders, poor social supports, domestic violence, financial concerns and/or reduced accessibility to services. Populations that have few economic, social or psychological resources to assist them to cope with ill-health are at risk of poorer health outcomes.

Poverty and social disadvantage are factors that have the single most devastating effect on specific groups in society, including females, the young and old, single parents, persons in regional areas, Aboriginal and Torres Strait Islander people, persons born in non-English speaking countries, persons in private rental accommodation, persons with a long-term health condition and persons who did not complete secondary school (or its equivalent) (McLachlan, Gilfillan & Gordon, 2013). Education is significant because, without it, populations limit their employment opportunities, lifestyle choices, skill development and capacity building for resilience. Poor or unsafe environments can influence the level of individual and population exposure to health risks. Further, limiting opportunities to make healthy lifestyle choices can be detrimental to the health of that population. The following statistics relating to poverty provide an Australian perspective, demonstrating clear differences between rural and regional, as well as metropolitan, opportunities.

- 2 265 000 people (12.8%) were living below the poverty line, i.e. one in eight persons
- 575 000 children (17.3%) were living below the poverty line, i.e. one in six children
- 63% of people in unemployed households were below the poverty line
- 25% of people in lone parent households were below the 50% poverty line
- 14% of women were below the poverty line compared with 12% of men
- 54% of people living in households below the poverty line were female compared with 46% male
- 26% of adults living in households below the 50% poverty line came from a non-English speaking country
- The level of poverty was higher (13.1%) outside capital cities than in capital cities (12.6%) (Australian Council of Social Service, 2012).

Useful website:

Australian Council of Social Service
http://www.acoss.org.au

There are demonstrated links between low income and poor child and adult outcomes, with children born into and growing up in poverty more likely to:

- be in poor health and have learning and behavioural difficulties
- show lower levels of achievement at school
- become pregnant at an early age
- have lower skills and aspirations
- be in low-paid work or unemployed and welfare dependent as adults (Brooks-Gunn & Duncan, 1997; Brooks-Gunn, Duncan & Maritato, 1997; Scutella & Smyth, 2005; McLachlan et al., 2013).

These data provide rural nurses and midwives with a platform for informing and assisting parents to make informed decisions about nutrition, immunisation, and safety and accessibility to services and resources, thereby creating opportunities to meet the health needs of the whole family.

Illicit drug use

Illicit drug use and over-the-counter poly-drug use is rife in women of reproductive age. While the Australian Government is committed to harm minimisation, society fluctuates between distain and support for this approach. Women who are pregnant and use illicit drugs are seen as challenging and can be cared for poorly, often stigmatised and marginalised (Miles, Francis & Chapman, 2010). Nurses and midwives are often charged with finding ways of working with these women and families. A recent qualitative study (Miles, 2013) examined and developed an understanding of the phenomenon of midwives' experiences of caring for pregnant women who use illicit drugs. Three fundamental themes were revealed: making a difference, establishing partnerships and letting go, and redefining practice.

Establishing partnerships with women who were vulnerable is one of the most important components of care, with partnerships being built on trust, honesty and understanding. This professional relationship enables the midwife to meet the individual needs of the women and engage other service providers to provide timely services. Working with women who use illicit drugs is very emotional work, with midwives expressing a range of emotions from love, anxiety, compassion, sadness to respect and admiration (Miles, Chapman & Francis, 2012). Health professionals need to expand their capacity to be resilient and to be able to bounce back, to be disappointed yet realistic in their expectations of others. Most importantly, they need to see the woman as a pregnant woman first, with drug use and other issues following.

Useful websites:

Australian Drug Information Network
http://www.adin.com.au

Women's Alcohol and Drug Service
http://www.thewomens.org.au/AlcoholDrugService

Adolescence and pregnancy

Adolescence is a time that has often been associated with increased risk-taking behaviours, including the use of drugs and alcohol as well as sexual activity. There are substantial health challenges for adolescent Australians, and more so in rural and remote areas, especially with the demonstrated and significantly higher rates of adolescent pregnancy. In 2011, 11 420 babies were born to adolescent women, a reduction of approximately 1.5% from 2008 (Australian Bureau of Statistics [ABS], 2012), and there are limited data on the amount of terminations. What is known is that there are far more adolescent women in rural and remote geographical areas of Australia giving birth than in the metropolitan areas. It is estimated that approximately one in every five adolescent women aged 15–20 years gets pregnant, with approximately one in every 10 women giving birth (Chan & Sage, 2005; Kirkman, Rowe, Hardiman & Rosenthal, 2011). A recent study focusing on young mothers' experiences found that they are more likely to be unemployed, live in poverty, give birth to low birth weight babies, encounter increased risks of accidents to their toddlers, have reduced access to health and social supports, and have poorer health outcomes (Roberts, Graham & Barter-Godfrey, 2011).

There are a number of noted suggestions from Australia (ABS) (http://www.abs.gov.au) and internationally (http://www.cdc.gov) to reduce the social and economic toll. These include improved sexual health education and access to confidential sexual health services, including the provision of contraception choices.

Useful websites:

Teenage pregnancy
http://www.betterhealth.vic.gov.au/bhcv2/bhcarticles.nsf/pages/Teenage_pregnancy

Parenting as a teenager
http://raisingchildren.net.au/articles/parenting_as_a_teenager.html/context/1000

Lily is a 16-year-old who is now 28 weeks' pregnant. She has attended the antenatal clinic for her glucose challenge test and while there tells you that she is unhappy at home. On further discussion she reveals to you that she lives with her 17-year-old boyfriend, who she has known for 8 months. In the house also lives her boyfriend's mother, his half siblings (with ages that range from 18 months to eight years) and the mother's new boyfriend, who moved into the house in the last month.

Lily tells you that she left school when she was 12 weeks' pregnant; she does not work. Her boyfriend, Justin, does not go to school either. He often goes out with his friends skateboarding and leaves her alone at his house. Lily has no contact with her own mum since she told her she was pregnant, and there was a big scene and she left and went to Justin's house. Her dad left the family when she was four years old and she has not heard from him since. She occasionally hears from her younger sister, Paris, who is 12. Lily does not drink alcohol but tells you that she does smoke marijuana most nights, as both she and Justin are supplied by the mother's boyfriend. Lily does not trust this man and feels uncomfortable when she is alone with him.

She becomes very teary, saying she feels trapped but has no alternative other than to stay where she is. She has nothing for the baby and does not know what she is going to do.

Questions

1 What priorities need to be worked on in the antenatal period (including social, emotional and physical)?
2 What are your decision-making rationales?

Mandatory reporting

Mandatory reporting is the legal requirement for suspected cases of child abuse and neglect. All local and national authorities have mandatory reporting requirements of some description. However, the people mandated to report and the abuse types for which it is mandatory to report vary across Australian states and territories (Higgins, Bromfield, Richardson, Holzer & Berlyn, 2010).

Nurses and midwives are included in the number of professionals (police, doctors, nurses and teachers) who are legally obliged to report suspected child abuse. If any of the above professionals become concerned that a child/young person known to them in their capacity as a mandatory reporter is being abused or neglected, or are at risk of being abused or neglected, they need to report their concerns to the Child Protection Helpline. These decisions are not always easy as the consequences are considerable.

Each Australian state and territory has its own significant procedures, and those who are mandated to report their concerns range from a limited number of specified persons in specified contexts (Queensland) through to every adult (Northern Territory). As health professionals, nurses need to increase their familiarity with these reporting processes in the state or territory in which they work (or study) to be able to report confidently within the parameters laid down by the relevant Acts and Regulations. It is important to keep in mind that those families who require child protection services are reported promptly. If possible, the concerns should also be discussed with the family; this may provide an opportunity to refer to other services or for a more appropriate service to become involved. However, this may not always be possible and sometimes may be detrimental to the child or family if there is risk of flight. For a nurse and midwife who lives in a rural or remote area, this process might be more difficult as both the health professional and family will be known in the community. Providing alternative options to the statutory child protection system for assistance to children, young people and families requires the health professionals to be involved in networks of community and community health care in their locality and those nearby (NSW Department of Community Services, 2010).

Useful website:

Australian Institute of Family Studies
http://www.aifs.gov.au/

Go to the search box and type **Mandatory reporting of child abuse and neglect** (access information for your state or territory).

Dying, death and bereavement

Fatal childhood illnesses in Australia are rare. It is estimated that approximately 16 per 10 000 children and adolescents aged 0–19 years may require palliative care services. Unlike their adult counterparts, only about 40% of these will have a diagnosis of cancer; the majority of dying children in Australia will succumb to congenital and genetic disorders and neuromuscular diseases (Monterosso & De Graves, 2012).

However, the AIHW reports that there is higher infant and child mortality in remote and rural areas than in regional and metropolitan areas (Queensland University of Technology/AIHW, 2004). It is very uncommon for a child in a rural community to die of natural causes; however, when the situation arises, the challenges facing rural families are specific to their geographical distance from specialist paediatric services. Through the illness trajectory, with a change in goals of care, and to death, many families rely upon the health services typically found in large metropolitan centres. Even Australia's largest regional cities rarely have services appropriate for the care of the dying child and their family. Clinical response to many life-threatening childhood illnesses is to pursue curative or life-prolonging treatment even until the death of the child; leukaemia is one example. Subsequently, it is not unusual that one parent stays with their child during their time in city-based healthcare services, while the other parent remains at home to work and care for their other children. This necessity bears with it a financial burden – perhaps already compromised by the loss of income via the accompanying parent; travel costs, parking, accommodation, food and other costs of daily living all add up over the duration of the child's illness.

However, it is more usual that a child will be brought home to die (Hynson & Drake, 2012). Caring for someone dying at home is known to be one of the most challenging undertakings (Palliative Care Australia, 2004), particularly when it is a child dying, and even more so when the child is dying within a community that is under-resourced and distant from specialist healthcare services. It is argued that the clinical and social needs of dying children and their families in rural settings are poorly understood by both clinicians and communities (Monterosso, Kristjanson, Auon & Phillips, 2007).

Two factors are imperative in facilitating the best possible levels of support and care at home for the dying child and their family:

- establish optimum communication between specialist care services and local clinicians to ensure an appropriate skill set is developed, and
- promote an acceptable level of involvement of the family's community in their support and care.

Communication between specialist services and local clinicians is not just a matter of a well-written discharge plan sent in a timely fashion! Local clinicians involved in the child's care should have the opportunity to discuss with the specialist service the goals of care, the palliative treatment strategies and the family's concerns. Increasingly, the technological means to provide assistance help bridge the distance between city and country and are an affordable and effective option if available (Smith, Bensink, Armfield, Stillman & Caffery, 2005). The palliative care of children involves uncommon medications or medications used in uncommon doses; subcutaneous infusions to control symptoms may be a key intervention. Sound information from the referring service about these clinical palliative care interventions is essential, and this may address some identified deficits for rural-based nurses (Rosenberg &

Canning, 2004). There are some excellent resources available in Australia; in particular, Monterosso and De Graves (2012) provide insights for the care of dying children, especially their *Developmental guidelines for assessment of symptoms in children* (pp. 366–7).

The value of mobilising local communities to support families with a dying child cannot be underestimated. As the compassionate response of a capable community (Kellehear & Young, 2011), this is frequently seen in rural communities during times of collective hardship such as bushfire, flood or mass trauma, such as that seen in the 2002 Bali bombings (Rosenberg, 2009). However, a community's capacity to support one of their own dying children varies enormously. The subject of death remains a source of discomfort for many and, like any community, there are alliances and conflicts in rural settings. Each family can be assisted to articulate their needs for support from their community (Kellehear, 2005). This may range from complete privacy through to a fully engaged network of supporters; whilst the latter *seems* best, it is ultimately a matter for each family to decide. This may take the form of practical support, shopping or meals, school transport for other children in the family or assistance with housework or yard care. Whilst there may be a family member or friend who undertakes coordination of this network of support, it may fall to the local community nurse or GP practice manager to organise.

The loss of a child is a known risk factor for complicated grieving (Lobb et al., 2010; Monterosso & De Graves, 2012). In developed countries, the death of a child is seen as an aberration to the normal course of events; the emotional and social isolation experienced by bereaved parents and siblings can be exacerbated by geographical isolation. The capacity of rural communities to provide appropriate support to bereaved families will vary and requires assessment. The role of the nurse providing palliative care to the dying child should include understanding the normal reactions to the loss of a child, the signs of complicated grieving and the communication of opportunities for ongoing family support.

Useful website:

Australian Centre for Grief and Bereavement
http://www.grief.org.au

Summary

In this chapter, we have discussed how:

- generalist rural nurses and midwives play a vital role in supporting maternal and child health in rural communities
- in many instances they provide first-line care in primary health care, community care and acute care
- alternatively, they provide the conduit to referral pathways to other members of the interdisciplinary team, with some located in the same community, others provided by outreach services, and still others located in larger regional centres
- rural nurses and midwives must meet the diverse needs of their rural communities, with each one having its own unique demographic
- the roles played by nurses and midwives cannot be underestimated, for the health and wellbeing of whole communities can be attributed to the professional competence of this workforce.

Reflective questions

1 What models of midwifery care are available in your community?
2 Why is it important for fathers to be involved in care provision for partners and children?
3 What are the major issues relating to child health in Australia?
4 What are the mandatory reporting requirements in your state/territory?
5 What does it mean to be disadvantaged?
6 How could you work more effectively with a woman who uses illicit drugs?

References

Aday, L. A. (1994). Health status of vulnerable populations. *Annual Review of Public Health*, 15(1), 487–509. doi: 10.1146/annurev.pu.15.050194.002415

Arora, A., Scott, J. A., Bhole, S., Do, L., Schwarz, E. & Blinkhorn, A. S. (2011). Early childhood feeding practices and dental caries in preschool children: A multi-centre birth cohort study. *BMC Public Health*, 11(1), 1–7. doi: 10.1186/1471–2458–11–28

Australian Bureau of Statistics (ABS). (2012). Number of teenage mothers lowest in a decade. Media release. Retrieved March 24, 2014, from www.abs.gov/ausstats/abs@.nsf/Latestproducts/3301.0Media%20Release12012?opendocument&tabname=Summary&prodno=3301.0&issue=2012&num=&view

Australian Council of Social Service. (2012). *Poverty in Australia Report,* ACOSS Paper 194. Sydney: ACOSS. Retrieved March 24, 2014, from http://acoss.org.au/uploads/ACOSS%20Poverty%20Report%202012_Final.pdf

Australian Institute of Health and Welfare (AIHW). (2012). *A picture of Australia's children 2012.* Cat. no. PHE 167. Canberra: AIHW. Retrieved March 24, 2014, from http://www.aihw.gov.au/WorkArea/DownloadAsset.aspx?id=10737423340

Barnes, M. & Rowe, J. (2009). *Child, youth and family health: Strengthening communities.* Sydney: Churchill Livingstone Australia.

Brooks-Gunn, J. & Duncan, G. J. (1997). The effects of poverty on children. *The Future of Children, Children and Poverty,* 7(2), 55–71.

Brooks-Gunn, J., Duncan, G. J. & Maritato, N. (1997). Poor families, poor outcomes: The well-being of children and youth. In G. J. Duncan & J. Brooks-Gunn (Eds.), *Consequences of growing up poor.* New York: Russell Sage Foundation.

Chan, A. & Sage, L. (2005). Estimating Australia's abortion rates (1985–2003). *The Medical Journal of Australia,* 182, 447–52.

Commonwealth of Australia. (2009). *Improving Maternity Services in Australia: The Report of the Maternity Services Review.* Canberra: Commonwealth of Australia.

Cox, J. L., Holden, J. M. & Sagovsky, R. (1987). Detection of postnatal depression: Development of the 10-item Edinburgh postnatal depression scale. *The British Journal of Psychiatry,* 150, 782–6. doi: 10.1192/bjp.150.6.782

Department of Health (DoH). (2012). *Maternal and infant health.* Canberra: Australian Government. Retrieved March 24, 2014, from http://www.health.gov.au/internet/main/publishing.nsf/Content/Maternal+and+Infant+Health-2

Department of Health and Ageing (DoHA). (2007). *The 2007 Australian National Children's Nutrition and Physical Activity Survey.* Canberra: Australian Government. Retrieved March 24, 2014, from http://www.health.gov.au/internet/main/publishing.nsf/Content/phd-nutrition-childrens-survey

Dietsch, E., Davies, C., Shackleton, P., Alston, M. & McLeod, M. (2008). *'Luckily we had a torch': Contemporary birthing experiences of women living in rural and remote NSW.* Wagga Wagga: School of Nursing and Midwifery, Faculty of Science, Charles Sturt University.

Eckermann, A., Dowd, T., Chong, E., Nixon, L., Gray, R. & Johnson, S. (2006). *Binan Goonj: Bridging cultures in Aboriginal health* (2nd ed.). Sydney: Churchill Livingstone Elsevier.

Elder, R., Evans, K. & Nizette, D. (2013). *Psychiatric and mental health nursing* (3rd ed.). Sydney: Mosby Elsevier.

Francis, K., McLeod, M. A., McIntyre, M., Mills, J. & Bradley, A. (2012). Australian rural maternity services: Creating a future or putting the last nail in the coffin. *Australian Journal of Rural Health,* 20, 281–4. doi: 10.1111/j.1440-1584.2012.013000.x

Glasper, A. & Richardson, J. (2010). *A textbook of children's and young people's nursing* (2nd ed.). Oxford, UK: Churchill Livingstone Elsevier.

Hazinski, M. F. (2013). *Nursing care of the critically ill child.* (3rd ed.) St Louis: Elsevier.

Higgins, D., Bromfield, L., Richardson, N., Holzer, P. & Berlyn, C. (2010). *Mandatory reporting of child abuse and neglect.* Melbourne: Commonwealth of Australia. Retrieved March 24, 2014, from www.aifs.gov.au

Homer, C., Brodie, P. & Leap, N. (2008). *Midwifery continuity of care.* Sydney: Churchill Livingstone Elsevier.

Hynson, J. & Drake, R. (2012). Paediatric palliative care in Australia and New Zealand. In C. Knapp, V. Madden & S. Fowler-Kerry (Eds.), *Pediatric palliative care: Global perspectives* (pp. 379–402). New York: Springer.

Kellehear, A. (2005). *Compassionate cities: Public health and end of life care.* London: Routledge.

Kellehear, A. & Young, B. (2011) Resilient communities. In S. Conway (Ed.), *Governing death and loss: Empowerment, involvement and participation* (pp. 89–98). Oxford, UK: Oxford University Press.

Kirkman, M., Rowe, H., Hardiman, A. & Rosenthal, D. (2011). Abortion is a difficult solution to a problem: A discursive analysis of interviews with women considering or undergoing abortion in Australia. *Women's Studies International Forum,* 34(2), 121–9. doi: http://dx.doi.org/10.1016/j.wsif.2010.11.002

Lobb, E. A., Kristjanson, L. J., Aoun, S. M., Monterosso, L., Halkett, G. K. B. & Davies, A. (2010). Predictors of complicated grief: A systematic review of empirical studies. *Death Studies,* 34(8), 673–98.

Lowdermilk, D. L., Perry, S. E., Cashion, K., Rhodes Alden, K. (2012). *Maternity & women's health care* (10th ed.). St Louis: Elsevier Mosby.

Macdonald, S. & Magill-Cuerden, J. (Eds.). (2011). *Mayes' midwifery* (14th ed.). Edinburgh: Bailliere Tindal Elsevier.

McLachlan, R., Gilfillan, G. & Gordon, J. (2013). *Deep and persistent disadvantage in Australia.* Melbourne, Vic: Productivity Commission. Retrieved March 24, 2014, from http://www.pc.gov.au/__data/assets/pdf_file/0007/124549/deep-persistent-disadvantage.pdf

McMurray, A. (2007). *Community health and wellness* (3rd ed.). Marrickville, NSW: Elsevier Australia.

Miles, M. (2013). Compassion, consequences and complexity – midwives' experiences of working with women who use illicit drugs. Paper presented at The National Nursing Forum: Success through Synergy. Canberra: Australian College of Nursing.

Miles, M., Chapman, Y. & Francis, K. (2012). Making a difference: The experiences of midwives working with women. *International Journal of Childbirth,* 2(4), 245–54. doi: http://dx.doi.org/10.1891/2156-5287.2.4.245

Miles, M., Francis, K. & Chapman, Y. (2010). Challenges for midwives: Pregnant women and illicit drug use. *Australian Journal of Advanced Nursing,* 28(1), 83–90.

Monterosso, L. & De Graves, S. (2012). Paediatric palliative care. In M. O'Connor, S. Lee & S. Aranda (Eds.), *Palliative care nursing: A guide to practice* (pp. 355–80). Ascot Vale: Ausmed.

Monterosso, L., Kristjanson, L. J., Auon, S. & Phillips, M. B. (2007). Supportive and palliative care needs of families of children with life-threatening illnesses in Western Australia: Evidence to guide the development of a palliative care service. *Palliative Medicine*, 21, 689–96.

NSW Department of Community Services. (2009). *Working with Aboriginal people and communities: A practice resource.* Sydney: DOCs. Retrieved March 24, 2014, from http://www.community.nsw.gov.au/docswr/_assets/main/documents/working_with_aboriginal.pdf

——. (2010). *The Structured Decision Making® System: New South Wales Mandatory Reporter Guide.* NSW, Australia: Children's Research Center. Retrieved March 24, 2014, from http://www.community.nsw.gov.au/kts/guidelines/documents/mandatory_reporter_guide.pdf

Pairman, S., Tracy, S., Thorogood, C. & Pincombe, J. (2010). *Midwifery preparation for practice.* Sydney: Churchill Livingstone.

Palliative Care Australia. (2004). *The hardest thing we have ever done – The social impact of caring for terminally ill people in Australia 2004: Full report of the national inquiry into the social impact of caring for terminally ill people.* Canberra: Palliative Care Australia.

Purrett, G. (2004). Calculating individualised due dates. In S. Wickham (Ed.), *Midwifery best practice 2.* Edinburgh: BFM Books for Midwives Elsevier.

Queensland University of Technology and the Australian Institute of Health and Welfare. (2004). *Health inequalities in Australia: Mortality.* Canberra: AIHW.

Reid-Searl, K., Dwyer, T., Moxham, L., Lovegrove, M. & Applegarth, J. (2012). *Nursing and midwifery: Student's clinical midwifery.* Frenchs Forest, NSW: Pearson.

Roberts, S., Graham, M. & Barter-Godfrey, S. (2011). Young mothers' lived experiences prior to becoming pregnant in rural Victoria: A phenomenological study. *Australian Journal Rural Health*, 19(6), 312–17. doi: 10.1111/j.1440-1584.2011.01228.x

Rosenberg, J. P. (2009). Circles in the surf: Australian masculinity, mortality and grief. *Critical Public Health*, 19(3–4), 417–26.

Rosenberg, J. P. & Canning, D. F. (2004). Palliative care by nurses in rural and remote practice. *Australian Journal of Rural Health*, 12(4), 166–71.

Scutella, R. & Smyth, P. (2005). *The Brotherhood's social barometer: Monitoring children's chances.* Melbourne: Brotherhood of St Laurence.

Smith, A. C., Bensink, M., Armfield, N., Stillman, J. & Caffery, L. (2005). Telemedicine and rural health care applications. *Journal of Postgraduate Medicine*, 51, 286–93.

6 Childhood and adolescence in rural communities

Ann-Marie Brown, Ainsley James and Angela Bradley

Learning objectives

On completion of this chapter, the reader will be able to:

- discuss the normal growth and development (developmental milestones) related to children in rural communities

- define and identify common health issues related to children and adolescents in rural communities, including respiratory disorders, injury/accidents and burns

- identify health promotion practices such as access to and application of appropriate screening tests as well as age-relevant immunisation requirements

- briefly discuss issues relating to mental and sexual health in relation to adolescence in rural communities

- describe and discuss access issues that children and adolescents in rural communities have in relation to accessing metropolitan health facilities.

Key words

Childhood conditions, mental health, adolescents, immunisation, growth and development

Chapter overview

This chapter provides a brief snapshot of children and adolescents in varying contexts of practice in rural environments. Common childhood conditions and aspects of adolescent health will be presented in conjunction with case studies and reflective questions to facilitate practical application.

Growth and development

Factors affecting growth and development fall into two main categories: heredity and genetic and environmental factors. In the early prenatal environment, the uterus shields the foetus from external adverse conditions, which may include maternal nutritional deficiencies, metabolic or endocrine disturbances, infectious diseases such as rubella, Rh incompatibility, smoking, alcohol and drugs. In the postnatal period, the environment determines the pace and pattern of growth and development. During this time, nutrition, infections, trauma, socioeconomic level, climate, cultural influences, emotional factors, chronic diseases and growth potentials will lay the groundwork for development of the child.

Although all babies and children have individual differences in their growth and development, certain milestones generally apply. Table 6.1 provides a snapshot of the typical growth and development of young children and adolescents.

TABLE 6.1 *Snapshot of typical growth and development of young children and adolescents.*

AGE OF CHILD	PHYSICAL ABILITIES	SPEECH/SOCIAL DEVELOPMENT	WEIGHT/HEIGHT
3 months	Reflexes disappear, stronger neck muscles. Able to turn head. Able to hold rattle. (Beckett & Taylor, 2010)	Oral development. Able to reach for objects. Able to differentiate cry: 'hunger', 'wet', 'lonely'. (Speedie, 2013)	Infants lose weight after birth but regain after 2–3 weeks. Weight gain 1.2 kg per month. (Speedie, 2013)
At the end of 3 months	Baby can raise head and chest when put on stomach. (Speedie, 2013)	Begins to make sounds such as cooing and vowel sounds. (Huberman, 2002)	Continues to increase weight at 1.2 kg per month. (Speedie, 2013)
4–6 months	Reflexes disappear; sits with support; begins to support body with legs when held in a standing position. (Beckett & Taylor, 2010)	Babbling and initiating sounds such as laughing and squealing with delight; blowing 'raspberries' and saying 'da', 'ma' and 'ba'. (Huberman, 2002)	As a rule, infants double their birth weight by 6 months. Height increases by 50% in first year. (Speedie, 2013)
7–9 months	Able to roll from their front to back, sits leaning forward at first, then sits unsupported. (Beckett & Taylor, 2010)	Double sounds such as 'da-da', 'ma-ma' and may also repeat tones and sounds made by others. Begins to say 'no'. (Huberman, 2002)	Weight gain approximately 600 g per month. (Speedie, 2013)
10–12 months	Pulls up into standing position, sits down again and walks supported by permanent objects such as furniture. Taking steps supported. (Beckett & Taylor, 2010)	Speech develops from 'da-da' and 'ma-ma' to knowing who these persons are. They may initiate sounds and some speech; shake their head for 'no'. (Huberman, 2002)	Child continues to grow approximately 600 g per month. (Speedie, 2013)

>>

»

1 year	Walks alone by 15 months and begins to run. Sits down on a stool or chair; climbs stairs while holding on and will dance to music. (Huberman, 2002)	Speech development increases, saying up to six simple words and 10–15 words at 18 months. Begins to say two-word sentences and imitates animal sounds and noises. Speech development by two years is generally 100 words or more. (Huberman, 2002)	Weight gain on average is about 227 g each month and birth weight triples by the end of the first year. Average height growth is about 0.64–1.27 cm each month. (Speedie, 2013)
2 years	They are very active, can run and throw and catch balls. They can stand on one foot; may like to climb on playground structures and ride a tricycle. (Huberman, 2002)	Their speech is becoming clearer and sentences are formed using 200–300 words. They begin to say small sentences. (Huberman, 2002)	Growth rate continues to slow. Average weight gain about 1.8–2.7 kg per year. Average height gain is 0.6–1.27 cm each month. (Beckett & Taylor, 2010)
3 years	Walks, runs, jumps easily, stands on tiptoe and rides a tricycle. (Gerhardt, 2005; Huberman, 2002)	Can speak 500–900 words and speaks in sentences of three to five words. A three-year-old will name colours, understand 'little' and 'big', 'yesterday' and 'tomorrow', and longer sentences. (Huberman, 2002)	Average weight gain is about 1.8–2.7 kg per year. Average height gain is 5–8 cm per year. (Huberman, 2002)
4–5 years	Develops more coordinated large motor skills, enabling them to skip, run and climb up and down stairs. Develops fine motor skills, enabling them to tie shoelaces, button shirts, use scissors and draw recognisable figures. (Gerhardt, 2005; Huberman, 2002)	They generally know 'good' and 'bad' and are able to follow rules. They understand and undertake simple activities to be healthy, such as brushing teeth or washing hands, and begin to understand privacy. (Gerhardt, 2005; Huberman, 2002)	Children of this age continue to grow but at a slower rate than during infancy and the toddler years. Some organs grow faster than the body, giving preschoolers a rounded tummy. They reach at least 50% of their adult height and about 20% of their adult weight by age five. (Gerhardt, 2005; Huberman, 2002)
6–8 years	They use small and large motor skills in sports and other activities. (Beckett & Taylor, 2010; Huberman, 2002)	Most children aged six to eight years will develop the skills to process more abstract concepts and complex ideas. They spend more time with the peer group and turn to peers for information. Friends and peer group become increasingly important. (Beckett & Taylor, 2010; Huberman, 2002)	Children at this age experience slower growth of about 6 cm in height and 4 kg in weight per year. They grow longer legs relative to their total height and begin resembling adults in the proportion of legs to body. They develop less fat and grow more muscle than in their earlier years. (Beckett & Taylor, 2010; Huberman, 2002)

»

》》

9–12 years	They become more independent and continue to develop decision-making skills and start to think about future careers and occupations. (Huberman, 2002)	Their peer group is greatly influential and there is an increased capability for social conscience and for abstract thought. At this age they may want to blend in and not stand out from their peers in any way, particularly as to gender roles and sexuality. (Beckett & Taylor, 2010)	Most young people aged nine to 12 years will experience a growth spurt with significant weight gain, muscle growth and genital maturation. This growth spurt begins earlier for girls and lasts longer for boys, who end up taller. (Beckett & Taylor, 2010)
13–17 years	They may seek increased power over their own lives and increase their independence. At this time many become risk takers and push the boundaries with their parental figures and teachers. (Gerhardt, 2005)	Most will achieve cognitive maturity with an ability to make decisions based on knowledge of options and their consequences. (Gerhardt, 2005)	This is a time of complete puberty and the physical transition from childhood to adulthood. Physically, they reach nearly their adult height, especially females. However, males continue to grow taller into their early 20s. (Beckett & Taylor, 2010; Huberman, 2002)
18 years and older	Fully understands abstract concepts and is generally aware of consequences and personal limitations. (Huberman, 2002)	Identifies career goals and prepares to achieve them. Secures their autonomy and builds and tests their decision-making skills. They may develop new skills, hobbies and adult interests. (Huberman, 2002)	Completes the process of physical maturation, usually attaining full adult height. (Huberman, 2002)

Childhood

Childhood is defined for this chapter as one month to 10 years of age. During this time of life, changes in growth and development occur: not only does the child grow heavier and taller, but the ability to perform skills and the development of thinking and socialising also alter greatly (Speedie, 2013). Surroundings and interaction with other individuals both impact on a child's health.

Issues surrounding childhood diseases in rural locations differ from those of the city, as access to health care and shortages of almost all health professionals and health-related infrastructure are important factors in overall health (see Chapters 1 and 2). The health status of younger people in rural areas is considerably worse than that of their city counterparts; also, the infant mortality rate is twice and three times that of Aboriginal and Torres Strait Islander Australians, respectively (Smith, 2007).

Many residents of the 1500 rural and remote communities that make up a third of Australia's population face significant health disadvantage and reduced access to health services (Australian Institute of Health and Welfare [AIHW], 2008). Research findings in Australia demonstrate that there is a critical work-force shortage in rural and remote communities. This shortage results in poor access to health care and lower health status of rural and remote area residents compared to urban residents (Doherty, 2007; Hemphill, Dunn, Barich & Infante, 2007; Liaw & Kilpatrick, 2008; Winters, Cudney & Sullivan, 2010). Delays of access and inferior coordination of services mean that problems are often compounded and that secondary complications arise, resulting in increased need for services. Thus a flow-on effect occurs as health professionals miss the opportunity to participate fully with families presenting with health issues (Wakerman et al., 2008).

Good health also supports child and adolescent development through some of the common problems of development, such as childhood illnesses, toilet training in young children, learning difficulties, sexuality, eating disorders and substance abuse for the adolescent (Huberman, 2002).

Common childhood disorders in rural Australia

Respiratory conditions

Asthma in Australia has a greater prevalence than in many countries world-wide (Asthma Australia, 2011–2012). In 2011–2012, 10.2% of Australians (or around 2.3 million people) had asthma. Overall, males and females reported similar rates of asthma (9.5% of males and 10.9% of females); however, rates of asthma across age groups show a different pattern (Australian Bureau of Statistics [ABS], 2013). Asthma is one of the most common childhood dis-orders in both rural and metropolitan regions of Australia. The prevalence of asthma (estimated from self-reported data from the 2007–2008 National Health Survey as part of the ABS) tends to be significantly higher in people living in areas with lower socioeconomic status (SES) than in people living in areas with higher SES. People living in rural areas often have a lower SES than those in metropolitan regions. The prevalence of asthma is also significantly higher in people living in inner regional areas than in those living in major cities (AIHW, 2011a).

Amongst children aged 0–14 years, males had a higher rate of asthma (11.4%) than did females (7.2%). However, from 15 years of age, asthma is more common in women than men (ABS, 2013). Hospitalisation rates for asthma are higher in rural areas than in metropolitan areas owing to access to health care and possible exposure to pollens, pesticides and chemicals (Victorian Department of Health, 2013).

The main causes of increased asthma rates in rural areas are strongly related to harvest and the number of pollens in the regions at particular times during the year. During harvest time, many particles and seeds become airborne and are inhaled, causing hay fever and asthma-like symptoms. Pesticides and herbicides used by farmers throughout seasonal spraying also increase the risk of asthma-like symptoms in rural areas, as does burning off paddocks after harvest. One of the major issues in these areas is that many children may never have had asthma but then develop asthma-like symptoms that require urgent medical treatment. Children already diagnosed with asthma often have an asthma management plan, which needs to be adhered to during exacerbations. Presentation to hospital is generally higher for the children who have not been previously diagnosed. At times, asthma management plans are not reviewed and may be out of date owing to lack of access to medical officers or asthma educators.

Aboriginal and Torres Strait Islander children have a greater incidence of asthma due to passive smoking before and after birth (Asthma Australia,

One rural hospital is closely linked with the local university. Owing to its location and the severity of asthma in the region, the university undertakes surveillance of the regional pollen count and thunderstorm alerts. The university is able to inform the local hospitals and (registered) patients by text of the increased pollen count or thunderstorm risk and therefore the increased risk of their asthma flaring up. Patients are advised to remain indoors or ensure their asthma management plan is up to date and that they have appropriate medication if they become unwell.

VIGNETTE

The local hospital's emergency department is then able to prepare for incoming patients, which may require increased numbers of nursing and other health professional staff. This is an excellent mechanism for alerting asthmatics to potential dangers, thus preventing major complications occurring.

Questions
1 Are you aware of any other collaborative initiatives that support the health and wellbeing of local communities?
2 If so, in your opinion, are these methods useful for harnessing local resources and improving health outcomes?
3 Why?

2007–2008). Moreover, Aboriginal and Torres Strait Islander children aged 0–14 years are more likely to attend hospital emergency departments with asthma in late February and have a higher rate of admission with asthma than non-Indigenous children and adults; this is higher in boys aged 0–4 years (Asthma Australia, 2007–2008). The access to follow-up and compliance with asthma management plans are also an issue for Aboriginal and Torres Strait Islander children. Aboriginal and Torres Strait Islander families may not have the resources required to manage their child/ren's asthma or they may live in isolated places, thus reducing their ability to utilise services. Asthma education is conducted in rural communities for Aboriginal and Torres Strait Islander children and parents to assist with compliance, use of medications and asthma management plans. Younger children are prone to developing bronchiolitis, croup and other respiratory illnesses that have asthma-type symptomatology.

Accidents and injuries

Young children in rural communities present to local health facilities with a wide range of injuries sustained from farming equipment and farm-related activities, sporting events, school and home injuries, motor vehicle accidents and poisonings, to name a few. The rates of hospitalisation due to injury or accidents are two to four times greater in rural than in metropolitan areas (Smith 2007; Stiller, Depczynski, Fragar & Franklin, 2008). Stiller et al. (2008) found that approximately 30 children aged 0–14 years die on Australian farms each year. Table 6.2 outlines the key injury risks on farms.

TABLE 6.2 *Key injury profile risks.*

Drowning of young children (0–5 years)
Injury associated with farm vehicles
Injury associated with farm machinery
Injury associated with two- and four-wheeled motorcycles (especially boys 5–14 years)
Horse-related injury (especially girls 10–14 years)

(Adapted from Stiller et al., 2008, p. 3).

Many rural children and adolescents live on farms and enjoy horseriding from a young age. Injuries resulting from falls while horseriding or being near uncontrolled horses can be serious. Spinal and facial fractures and internal injuries from horse-related accidents often require children to be airlifted to major metropolitan trauma centres for assessment and management. Not all rural hospitals have medical personnel able to assess a child appropriately. Limited access to medical imaging and pathology laboratories can compromise health outcomes. The longer it takes to transport an injured child to a hospital, the more likely the risk of developing serious complications or death.

Major regional hospitals provide outreach assistance to smaller health facilities, including assessing patients over the phone or via videoconferencing or telemedicine technologies (Moffatt & Eley, 2010). Highly qualified medical and nursing staff are able to support local nurses and doctors to instigate effective management strategies and, if required, to assist in stabilising the child for transfer to a hospital for specialist care. This model of care is commonly adopted, ensuring that small rural health facilities have access to specialist medical, nursing, midwifery and allied health professionals, albeit at a distance.

Motorbike and quad (four-wheel) bike accidents and injuries involving children are common in rural areas, as many children use them for work and recreation. In 2011, there were 18 deaths attributed to quad bike accidents in rural areas (Farmsafe Australia, 2013). Quad bike accidents are the leading cause of death in rural communities. The numbers are higher among children aged more than 15 years but are also significant in young children, who are often passengers on quad bikes and either fall off or are run over because of the instability of the bike on uneven ground. Often, as passengers, these children are unrestrained and may not have helmet protection.

Injuries from quad bikes and motorbikes range from simple fractures to major head and spinal injuries and, often, internal injuries. These injuries take a great deal of time to heal and need to be managed initially at a major trauma hospital; follow-up measures include rehabilitation, which can last for many months.

Contact burns and flame injuries occur more frequently in rural children than in children who reside in urban areas. It is recommended that any education campaign targeting childhood injuries considers these differences (Hyland, Zeni, Harvey & Holland, 2013). Injuries frequently occur in garages/sheds, farms, bush and forests (Hyland et al., 2013). Toddlers are the most vulnerable childhood group and are most at risk of being scalded. It is a common pastime for rural Australians to go camping or spend time around the campfire with friends and family. Young children left unsupervised are at risk of tripping over hot water or falling into the fire.

Although scald burns from hot drinks are the most common cause of burns admissions in children in high-income countries, the most common cause of burns injury requiring admission to a rural health facility in 2011–2012 was contact burns from hot ash (Martin, 2013). This rate increases when children are visiting from metropolitan regions. Further, children of lower SES are at greater risk of sustaining a burns injury. Burns in the Aboriginal and Torres Strait Islander community are three times greater than in the Caucasian community and also account for over 50% of all burns (*How to treat burns*, 2006). Burns injuries in rural communities are seen with farming equipment and motorbikes and are classified as contact with flames. These are more common than in metropolitan areas, where the most common burns are scalds (NSW Agency for Clinical Innovation [ACI], 2011).

Rural hospitals generally manage the initial care of children presenting with burns, which may involve resuscitation and preparation for transfer to a major trauma centre. Early first aid, pain management and fluid resuscitation are key to a good outcome with burns patients (NSW ACI, 2011). Initial management and preparation of the burnt areas for transfer depend on the receiving hospital. The length of time for retrieval will hinge on the severity of the burns. Often parents are expected to drive their child a number of hours to have a dressing reviewed or to see a consultant regarding smaller burns. The rural hospital can send the metropolitan hospital emails and photographs to aid initial assessment and to determine the need for transfer (NSW ACI, 2011).

Most of the injuries discussed are preventable. With this in mind, a task force was formed by Farmsafe Australia in 2008 inviting parents, farmers, and government and injury experts to discuss prevention strategies that would help rural families avoid injury to children on their properties (Stiller et al., 2008). One of the major issues is that families working on farms can be lax in supervising children, allowing them to play on farming equipment whilst their parents work (Stiller et al., 2008). Basic outcomes from the task force included the use of helmets whilst riding and seatbelts in vehicles, and preventing young children riding on the back of tractors and quad bikes (Stiller et al., 2008).

Other childhood issues

Children in rural areas suffer from the usual childhood conditions, including fractures, appendicitis and infections such as gastroenteritis, with prevalence rates similar to those of children in metropolitan regions. The main issue is a lack of specialist care for children in a number of rural areas. Many of the rural hospitals have visiting or locum (casual) medical staff who may not be experienced in managing and treating children. These locums come from various regions and are possibly recruited from overseas, with very limited knowledge of children or local issues. Rural areas have difficulty attracting and keeping permanent medical staff.

Many rural hospitals do not have medical officers available after hours or on weekends, and this requires assessment of children to be undertaken by nursing staff who may or may not have the requisite knowledge and skills. Transferring children to more specialised healthcare services can involve travelling long distances, which can impact adversely on health outcomes and potentially be financially burdensome on parents and the transferring health service (Hegney, 2007). Monetary assistance is occasionally available for travel costs, but this is often not enough to cover accommodation and meals during the stay at a metropolitan hospital (Hegney, 2007). Also, long-distance travel increases the risk of fatigue and motor vehicle accidents due to high-speed driving (Hegney, 2007).

Children in rural areas have higher rates of dental caries than children living in metropolitan areas. Rural children have twice as many caries and are four times more likely to be hospitalised and require general anaesthetic to treat decay than children who live in metropolitan areas (Gussy, Waters & Kilpatrick, 2006). Preschool children living in rural areas have significantly less access to dental health programs than children who live in metropolitan areas. The lack of consistent dental services for rural communities contributes to poor oral health and overall health status. Even when dental services are locally available, the cost of these services is often prohibitive, further contributing to health inequity experienced by rural children and their families.

Olivia, a four-year-old child of Aboriginal descent, was camping with her family during winter at a local river. As a normal routine, the family had lit a small fire around which to gather and chat about the events of the day. A 'billy' was on the fire; Olivia and her older brother were playing around the fire when Olivia tripped, and the hot water from the billy spilt all over her legs. Olivia was screaming in pain and her parents swiftly removed her track pants and applied cold water. They quickly drove her to the local hospital, which was two hours away. On arrival, the child was crying in pain and both her legs were red from her ankles to her upper thighs. The burns were circumferential, and blisters were appearing on her upper right thigh and both ankles. Her genital region was not involved.

Intranasal fentanyl was administered on arrival and an intravenous (IV) cannula was inserted. IV fluids were commenced and the burns were assessed. The child was further cooled with water to her legs and was readied for transfer to a

VIGNETTE

》 metropolitan children's hospital. Glad wrap was applied to both legs, as per the burns protocol, and air transport was organised. The parents were informed of the treatment and transfer, and they made their own arrangements and decided who was going to go with Olivia.

Olivia was transferred and spent five days in a burns unit in a major children's hospital. Her mother went with her in the air ambulance and her father was left to mind the other five children. She returned to her rural hospital and continued to receive dressings as an outpatient. Olivia required follow-up for three months, with dressings undertaken daily to second daily for the first month and then twice weekly.

Questions
Discuss the following implications for Olivia and her family in relation to transfer to a metropolitan health facility:
- effect on family
- separation anxiety for the child
- follow-up requirements – dressings/medications/further surgery
- cost to family
- long-term management of burns – scarring/garments/surgery
- immunisation requirements for children
- education for parents regarding long-term effects of burns in children
- cultural sensitivity related to Olivia's Aboriginal background
- analgesia and possible effects on Olivia if used over a long period of time.

Immunisation

Owing to the success of immunisation programs, many of the infectious diseases once prevalent in society no longer exist. This eradication could also account for complacency amongst members and groups within society, leading to variations in immunity status across regions, for example in smaller geographical areas. The National Health Performance Authority (2013) published a report, *Healthy communities: Immunisation rates for children in 2011–12*, on the percentage of children who were considered fully immunised at one year, two years and five years of age in 2011–2012 by the 61 areas covered by the new network of Medicare Locals, as well as by about 325 smaller geographical units. The report noted that vaccine coverage rates were lower among five-year-olds than at other ages; the percentage of Aboriginal and Torres Strait Islander children fully immunised was lower than for other children, especially at one and five years of age; and some Medicare Local areas contained more than 1000 children aged one year, two years and five years of age who were not fully immunised.

While there are no specific references to immunisation for rural communities, the Australian Government Department of Health's *Immunise Australia Program* (2013) identifies that Aboriginal and Torres Strait Islander children living in certain regions require extra protection against some diseases, in particular invasive pneumococcal disease, which may present as pneumonia, meningitis, blood poisoning and/or ear infections such as otitis media. It is recommended that Aboriginal and Torres Strait Islander children have their risk and vaccination status for hepatitis B reviewed and be offered testing for previous hepatitis B infection and thereafter vaccination if non-immune. A booster dose of pneumococcal disease 10-valent (10vPCV and 13vPCV) is recommended at 12–18 months of age that replaces the booster dose of 23vPPV at 18–24 months of age in the Northern Territory, South Australia and Western Australia (Australian Government Department of Health and Ageing, 2013a).

The Australian Government provides a free hepatitis A vaccine to all Aboriginal and Torres Strait Islander children less than five years of age who live in Queensland, the Northern Territory, South Australia and Western Australia, as there is a high incidence of this disease in these jurisdictions. In the Northern Territory and some remote areas of South Australia, Hib PRP-OMP (a specific type of Hib [Haemophilus influenzae type b]) is recommended to be given to Aboriginal and Torres Strait Islander children at two, four and 12 months of age at the same time as their other vaccinations owing to the increased risk. The National School-based HPV (Human Papillomavirus) Vaccination Program provided as part of the National Immunisation Program is offered to Aboriginal and Torres Strait Islander males aged 12–13 years and 14–15 years, and to Aboriginal and Torres Strait Islander females aged 12–13 years (Australian Government Department of Health and Ageing, 2013b). See the following web link for the current immunisation schedule from the *Immunise Australia Program* (Australian Government Department of Health, 2013):

<http://www.health.gov.au/internet/immunise/publishing.nsf/Content/4CB9 20F0D49C61F1CA257B2600828523/$File/nips-oct2013.pdf>

Adolescence

Adolescence is a stage of transition from being a child to becoming a young adult and can be exciting, challenging, rewarding and tumultuous. There are varying definitions for adolescence and adolescents. For our purposes, adolescents are those aged 10–19 years, with the broader definition of young people including those aged 15–24 years (World Health Organization [WHO], 2012); adolescents and young people will be used interchangeably in this chapter. Adolescence is not unique to rural communities; the experiences rural adolescents undergo are, however. Some of the experiences unique to rural young people include issues related to mental health, sexuality, sexual health and health behaviours.

Mental health

According to McNamara (2012), youth mental health in rural communities, specifically that of adolescents and young adult males, is a concern and has been identified as a high priority. Campo (2009, as cited in McNamara, 2012) reported a number of factors that can increase suicide risk especially amongst young Australian males in rural communities. These factors included risk-taking behaviour, recreational boredom, poor mental health literacy in families and communities, and a reluctance to seek assistance for mental health issues or social support. On the contrary, a factor that appears to promote a resilient adolescent population is self-efficacy. Adolescents who have educational and recreational success, positive social experiences and transition to social and emotional responsibilities of early adulthood tend to hold high levels of self-efficacy (McNamara, 2012).

Living in rural communities can have an impact on the mental health of adolescents as they deal with the many aspects of and influences on their lives. One aspect of living in a rural or even remote community is the surrounding environment, specifically adolescents living on farming properties and experiencing challenges associated with farming the land. Prolonged drought in rural and remote areas is harmful to the mental health of young people and is compounded by the difficulty in accessing relief services (Carnie, Berry, Blinkhorn & Hart, 2011). Carnie et al. (2011) reported that young people affected by drought described experiencing difficulties with their mental health and relationships, both in the home and at school, and concern about their family, community, future, money and isolation. Young people in this study were torn between wanting to stay in school to give themselves the best long-term opportunities for their future and leaving school to return to working on the farm to support their family. These circumstances created feelings of being overwhelmed and anxious (Carnie et al., 2011). More detailed discussions on mental health in rural communities can be found in Chapter 9.

Sexuality, sexual health and health behaviours

Adolescence is a time of great change, growth and development. The young person experiencing the milestone of adolescence is searching for who they are, their identity and where they 'fit in' to their family, peer groups and community. Some young people move through this stage in their life without impact; however, there are others who struggle. One aspect that impacts on rural young people is that of sexuality or sexual identity. A young person's sexuality or sexual identity is how they see themselves regardless of their sex or biology. Biological identity relates to chromosomal sex characteristics, where gender identity relates to how the young person sees themselves or has a sense of 'who' they are as a male or female (Dietsch & Davies, 2013).

Warr and Hillier (1997) examined sexual health issues for young rural people living in a small town that was described as having a sense of security and being familiar and reassuring, but that was monotonous and predictable. Rural communities also tend to have less privacy as many residents know each other, with this lack of privacy potentially impacting on the management of adolescents' sexual health needs. Accessing health care, specifically related to sexual health, can be difficult, awkward and at times embarrassing for an adolescent. A friend's mother may work at the local health clinic or the local pharmacist may be a family member.

Adolescents are concerned about being seen while accessing health care and information, including purchasing condoms, because they perceive that there may be confidentiality issues whereby friends, family members or friends of parents are the ones to assist the young person (Warr & Hillier, 1997). Warr and Hillier (1997) identified that young female adolescents who purchase or carry condoms may be seen as having a bad reputation in addition to the embarrassment of making the purchase. This outcome may cause adolescents to forego the condoms or health care altogether and possibly compromise their sexual health practices rather than experience the potential embarrassment or anxiety. A result of such choices or behaviour is the risk of sexually transmitted infections and also teenage pregnancy.

Roberts, Graham and Barter-Godfrey (2011) explored young rural mothers' lived experiences prior to becoming pregnant and identified that rural adolescents need additional support services and relevant recreational activities as a method of discouraging risk-taking behaviour, which in turn could reduce the chance of pregnancy.

The young mothers in this study suggested a number of recommendations that could assist adolescents living in rural communities:

- the need for more recreational activities for young adolescents to reduce boredom and risk-taking behaviours
- the need for confidential youth services

- sexual health information to include real-life experiences from young people to increase engagement
- adolescents want more understanding, less judgement and for adults to be less authoritarian (Roberts et al., 2011).

Health behaviours are developed during adolescence and may be influenced by a number of factors, which in turn influence their behaviours in the long term (Bourke, Humphreys & Lukaitis, 2009). The health behaviours – related to diet, exercise, smoking and alcohol consumption – appeared to be interrelated. Young people who were more social tended to be the ones who participated in sport and consumed alcohol, while those who did not, but who also smoked, tended to be socially excluded (Bourke et al., 2009). Bourke et al. (2009) identified the interrelatedness of the social and rural context as influencing the health behaviours of adolescents and the level of influence on these health behaviours by the individual, family, community and society. They point out that 'level of influence' has a number of predisposing, enabling and reinforcing factors that further influence the health behaviours of adolescents in a rural community, insofar as these factors are either already present, support the behaviour or allow the behaviour to continue (Bourke et al., 2009).

Aboriginal and Torres Strait Islander Australians

According to the *Young Australians: Their health and wellbeing* 2011 report (AIHW, 2011b), many young Australians are faring very well; however, there are some areas of concern particularly among Aboriginal and Torres Strait Islander young people. However, there have been some positive changes in recent years, such as a significant decline in death by injury, asthma hospitalisations, notifications for hepatitis A, B and C, and improved survival for cancer – with a very high improvement in melanoma survival rates. There has been a decline in teenage pregnancies and smoking and illicit substance abuse, and improvements in national minimal standards for education and crisis intervention. Areas of concern continue to be diabetes, sexually transmissible infections and high rates of mental health disorders, as well as road accident deaths particularly among males living in remote areas.

The health and welfare of Australia's Aboriginal and Torres Strait Islander people report (AIHW, 2011c) cited a number of findings that significantly impact on the growth and development of Aboriginal and Torres Strait Islander people. In 2009, the total fertility rate for Aboriginal and Torres Strait Islander women was 2.6 babies compared with 1.9 for all women in Australia. Motherhood during the teenage years was much more common among Aboriginal and Torres Strait Islander girls (21% compared with 4% of all births in 2009). Babies born in 2005–2007 to Aboriginal and Torres Strait Islander mothers were twice as likely to be of low birth weight as babies born to other Australian mothers. The Aboriginal and Torres Strait Islander infant mortality rate declined between 1991 and 2008, although it remains twice that of non-Indigenous infants.

Aboriginal and Torres Strait Islander children aged 0–14 years are far more likely to be disadvantaged across a broad range of health, community and socioeconomic indicators compared with non-Indigenous young people. They are twice as likely to die from all causes (six times as likely from assault and four times as likely from suicide).

The hospitalisation rate for assault on Aboriginal and Torres Strait Islander children in 2008 was more than five times the rate for non-Indigenous children. Aboriginal and Torres Strait Islander children were hospitalised for burns and scalds at twice the rate of other children. They are six to seven times more likely to be in child protection services. Assault was the most common cause of hospitalisation for Aboriginal and Torres Strait Islander young people. They are also six times more likely to be teenage mothers, three times more likely to live in overcrowded housing, two to three times as likely to be daily smokers, and 15 times more likely to be in juvenile justice supervision or in prison. Nearly 12% of Aboriginal and Torres Strait Islander children who received a Child Health Check on or before 30 June 2009 had chronic suppurative otitis media; this is more than three times the rate accepted by the WHO and is classed as a significant health problem.

In 2008, almost one-third of Aboriginal and Torres Strait Islander young people (aged 16–24 years) had high or very high levels of psychological distress, which is more than twice the rate of non-Indigenous young Australians. Aboriginal and Torres Strait Islander young people were hospitalised more commonly for mental health and behavioural disorders at 1.8 times the non-Indigenous rate. The leading causes were schizophrenia, alcohol misuse and reactions to severe stress. Aboriginal and Torres Strait Islander young people die at a rate 2.5 times higher than that of non-Indigenous young people. Young people living in remote areas, whether Aboriginal and Torres Strait Islander or non-Indigenous, have higher death rates, more dental decay, are less likely to meet minimum standards for reading, writing and numeracy, and are more likely to be in jobless families and live in overcrowded conditions (AIHW, 2011c).

Summary

In this chapter, we have discussed how:

- children and adolescents in rural communities have difficulty accessing major hospitals, causing a great amount of stress and anxiety to parents
- injuries and accidents involving adolescents and children in rural areas are directly related to farming and livestock
- children in rural communities have a greater chance of being diagnosed with asthma or respiratory conditions than metropolitan-based children; Aboriginal and Torres Strait Islander children have an even greater risk
- mental health issues in adolescents in rural communities are directly related to working the land and poor access to mental health services
- rural families are less likely to seek assistance for their children and adolescents with mental health disorders.

Reflective questions

1 An adolescent couple have decided to have sexual intercourse. They are unsure of what protection they should use. They are also concerned, as they know some of the staff in the local pharmacy and supermarket. What information would you provide them?

2 A 16-year-old female you are caring for in an outpatient clinic thinks she may be pregnant after having unprotected sex a couple of months ago with a male she met at a party. She is scared that her parents will find out and doesn't know what to do next. You know she needs to see her GP but you also know her aunty is the receptionist at the medical clinic. How do you support this adolescent?

3 You are asked to visit the local secondary school to facilitate a health promotion session with the senior students (Years 11 and 12). Bearing in mind the risk-taking behaviour of adolescents, what health promotion activities would be relevant to this age group? How would you get them actively involved in the session?

4 A young mother presents to the local emergency department stating her three-year-old child, David, has had some difficulty breathing. David lives on a farm 40 minutes from the local town, which has mainly crop and sheep grazing. On examination, you identify David as having acute asthma and administer the appropriate treatment per the medical officer's orders. David

is admitted to hospital. On discharge, the nurse needs to educate David's mother regarding medications and early warning signs. How would the nurse conduct this session?

5 A 16-year-old Aboriginal and Torres Strait Islander young adult presents to the local health clinic with her two-month-old baby requesting immunisation. She states that she has no money to pay for immunisation as her partner left her on her own with no money. She doesn't really have any family as she lives on an outback property and works in a kitchen. The baby is clean but you discover she has terrible nappy rash. What advice can you give this young woman regarding immunisation and care for this baby?

Ross, a 17-year-old young man living on a rural property with his single mother, during winter decided to stoke the fire overnight as the weather conditions had been quite cold. His mother went to bed early as she has emphysema after many years of smoking. Ross stoked the fire up. The house they lived in was small and run-down as Ross was only working part time at the local takeaway shop and his mother was too unwell to complete any maintenance.

VIGNETTE

There were many empty cans in the house, including deodorant cans lying around on the floor. The wood used for the fire had a number of splinters and one of the splinters pierced the deodorant can, causing the contents to light up and spray all over the room. Ross was directly in front of the fire and his face, hair and clothing caught alight. He was able to remove the large jacket he had on and put the fire out.

Ross arrived at the local emergency department after being driven in by his mother. He had burns to his forehead, face, neck and chest. Blisters had developed on his face and neck. He was able to talk in full sentences but had black around his mouth and was beginning to have a hoarse voice.

The rural hospital placed IV cannula x 2 and IV fluids and discussed the management. Analgesia was administered, Ross was intubated to protect his airway as the rural hospital was unable to look after a patient in this condition. After intubation, contact was made with a major referral hospital, and he was flown by fixed-wing aircraft for further management. Paraffin was applied to the burnt area of his face, and his chest was covered with approved dressings. The referral hospital required specific dressings in preparation for review and early management. Glad wrap was placed around his arms.

Ross was flown to a burns unit and remained ventilated for two days. He was discharged in the following three days and required continual follow-up with the burns unit and local hospital.

Questions
Discuss the following implications on the child/adolescent for the transfer of patients to large city hospitals:
- effect on family
- follow-up requirements – dressings/medications/further surgery
- cost of employment, hospital stay
- long-term management of burns – scarring/garments/surgery
- immunisation requirements for adolescents
- education for adolescents regarding risk-taking behaviours
- psychological effects of scarring on teenagers.

References

Asthma Australia. (2007–2008). Statistics. Retrieved March 24, 2014, from www. asthmaaustralia.org.au/Statistics.aspx

———. (2011–2012). What is asthma? Retrieved March 24, 2014, from http://www. asthmaaustralia.org.au/Statistics.aspx

Australian Bureau of Statistics (ABS). (2013). 4338.0 – *Profiles of Health, Australia, 2011–13. Asthma.* Retrieved March 24, 2014, from http://www.abs.gov.au/ ausstats/abs@.nsf/Lookup/4338.0main+features152011–13

Australian Government Department of Health. (2013). *Immunise Australia Program.* Retrieved March 24, 2014, from www.health.gov.au/internet/immunise/ publishing.nsf/Content/history-of-ia-prog

Australian Government Department of Health and Ageing. (2013a). *The Australian Immunisation Handbook* (10th ed.). Canberra: Australian Government Department of Health and Ageing. Retrieved March 24, 2014, from http://www.immunise. health.gov.au/internet/immunise/publishing.nsf/Content/Handbook10-home

———. (2013b). *Myths and realities: Responding to arguments against vaccination. A guide for providers* (5th ed.). Retrieved March 24, 2014, from http://www.health. gov.au/internet/immunise/publishing.nsf/Content/1FC63A2886238E6CCA257 5BD001C80DC/$File/full-publication-myths-and-realities-5th-ed-2013.pdf

Australian Institute of Health and Welfare (AIHW). (2008). *Rural, regional and remote health: Indicators of health status and determinants of health.* AIHW Cat. No. PHE 97; Rural Health Series No. 9. Canberra: AIHW. Retrieved March 24, 2014, from http://www.aihw.gov.au/WorkArea/DownloadAsset. aspx?id=6442459831

———. (2011a). *Asthma in Australia 2011.* Retrieved March 24, 2104, from http:// www.aihw.gov.au/WorkArea/DownloadAsset.aspx?id=60129544677

———. (2011b). *Young Australians: Their health and wellbeing.* Cat. no. PHE 140. Canberra: AIHW. Retrieved March 24, 2014, from www.aihw.gov.au/WorkArea/ DownloadAsset.aspx?id=10737419259

———. (2011c). *The health and welfare of Australia's Aboriginal and Torres Strait Islander people, an overview 2011.* Cat. no. IHW 42. Canberra: AIHW. Retrieved March 24, 2014, from http://www.aihw.gov.au/WorkArea/DownloadAsset. aspx?id=10737418955

Beckett, C. & Taylor, H. (2010). *Human growth and development* (2nd ed.). London: Sage.

Bourke, L., Humphreys, J. & Lukaitis, F. (2009). Health behaviours of young, rural residents: A case study. *Australian Journal of Rural Health*, 17(2), 86–91. doi: 10.1111/j.1440–1584.2008.01022.x

Carnie, T., Berry, H., Blinkhorn, S. & Hart, C. (2011). In their own words: Young people's mental health in drought-affected rural and remote NSW. *Australian Journal of Rural Health*, 19(5), 244–8. doi: 10.1111/j.1440–1548.2011.01224.x

Dietsch, E. & Davies, C. (2013). The nursing role in reproductive and sexual health. In C. Haley (Ed.), *Pillitteri's child and family health nursing in Australia and New Zealand* (pp. 49–62). Sydney: Lippincott Williams & Wilkins.

Doherty, S. R. (2007). Could we care for Amillia in rural Australia? *Rural and Remote Health*, 7(4), 768.

Farmsafe Australia. (2013). *Quad bike safety*. Moree: Farmsafe Australia Inc. Retrieved March 24, 2014, from www.farmsafe.org.au/index.php?article=content/for.../quadbike

Gerhardt, S. (2005). *Why love matters: How affection shapes a baby's brain development*. London: Taylor & Francis.

Gussy, M. G., Waters, E. & Kilpatrick, N. M. (2006). A qualitative study exploring barriers to a model of shared care for pre-school children's oral health. *British Dental Journal*, 201, 165–70.

Hegney, D. (2007). Practice nursing in rural Australia. *Contemporary Nurse*, 26(1), 74–82.

Hemphill, E., Dunn, S., Barich, H. & Infante, R. (2007). Recruitment and retention of rural general practitioners: A marketing approach reveals new possibilities. *Australian Journal of Rural health*, 15, 360–7.

How to treat burns: Assessment and triage. (2006). *Australian Rural Doctor*, 17–20. Retrieved March 24, 2014, from http://www.rhef.com.au/wp-content/uploads/rural-doctor-how-to-treat-july06.pdf

Huberman, B. (2002). Advocates for youth. Retrieved March 24, 2014, from http://www.advocatesforyouth.org/topics-issues

Hyland, E., Zeni, G., Harvey, J. & Holland, A. (2013, October). Rural and metropolitan paediatric burns in NSW: A retrospective epidemiological analysis. Paper presented at the Australian and New Zealand Burn Association 37th Annual Scientific Meeting, Perth. Retrieved March 24, 2014, from http://events.cdesign.com.au/ei/viewpdf.esp?id=378&file=//srv3/events/eventwin/docs/pdf/anzba2013asm1abstract00100.pdf

Liaw, S. & Kilpatrick, S. (2008). *A textbook of Australian rural health*. Canberra: Australian Rural Health Education Network.

Martin, L. (2013, November). Paediatric hot ash burns to feet: Risk factors in Western Australia. Paper presented at the 11th Australasian Injury Prevention & Safety Promotion Conference, Fremantle, Western Australia. Retrieved March 24, 2014, from http://www.injuryprevention2013.com.au/paediatric-hot-ash-burns-to-feet-risk-factors-in-western-australia/

McNamara, P. M. (2012). Adolescent suicide in Australia: Rates, risk and resilience. *Clinical Child Psychology and Psychiatry*, 18(3), 351–69. doi: 10.1177/1359104512455812

Moffatt, J. & Eley, D. (2010). The reported benefits of telehealth for rural Australians. *Australian Health Review*, 34(3), 276–81. doi:10.1071/AH09794

National Health Performance Authority. (2013). *Healthy communities: Immunisation rates for children in 2011–12*. Sydney: National Health Performance Authority. Retrieved March 24, 2014, from http://www.nhpa.gov.au/internet/nhpa/publishing.nsf/Content/Healthy-communities/$file/HC_ImmRates_2011-12_FINAL_130409.pdf

NSW Agency for Clinical Innovation. (2011). *Clinical practice guidelines: Burn patient management*. Chatswood, NSW: ACI. Retrieved March 24, 2014, from http://www.aci.health.nsw.gov.au/__data/assets/pdf_file/0019/162631/Clinical_Practice_Guidelines_2012.pdf

Roberts, S., Graham, M. & Barter-Godfrey, S. (2011). Young mothers' lived experiences prior to becoming pregnant in rural Victoria: A phenomenological study. *Australian Journal of Rural Health*, 19(6), 312–17. doi:10.1111/j.1440-1584.2011.01228.x

Smith, J. (2007). *Australia's rural and remote health: A social justice perspective* (2nd ed.). Croydon, Vic: Tertiary Press.

Speedie, L. (2013). Principles of growth and development. In C. Haley (Ed.), *Pillitteri's child and family health nursing in Australia and New Zealand* (pp. 453–68). Sydney: Lippincott Williams & Wilkins.

Stiller, L., Depczynski, J., Fragar, L. & Franklin, R. (2008). An evidence-consultation base for developing child injury prevention priorities for Australian farms. *Health Promotion Journal of Australia*, 19(2), 91–6.

Victorian Department of Health. (2013). Asthma – National Health Priority Areas background paper. Melbourne: Victorian Department of Health. Retrieved March 24, 2014, from http://www.health.vic.gov.au/nhpa/asth-back.htm

Wakerman, J., Humphrey, J., Wells, R., Kuipers, P., Entwhistle, P. & Jones, J. (2008). Primary health care delivery models in rural and remote Australia – a systematic review. *BMC Health Services Research*, 8(276). doi: 10.1186/1472-6963-8-276

Warr, D. & Hillier, L. (1997). 'That's the problem with living in a small town': Privacy and sexual health issues for young rural people. *The Australian Journal of Rural Health*, 5(3), 132–9. doi: 10.1111/j.1440-1584.1997.tb00254.x

Winters, C., Cudney, S. & Sullivan, T. (2010). Expressions of depression in rural women with chronic illness. *Rural and Remote Health*, 10, 1533 (Online). Retrieved March 24, 2014, from http://www.rrh.org.au/publishedarticles/article_print_1533.pdf

World Health Organization (WHO). (2012). *Adolescent health*. Geneva: WHO. Retrieved March 24, 2014, from http://www.who.int/topics/adolescent_health/en/

7 Working with adults in rural communities

Ysanne Chapman and Karen Francis

Learning objectives On completion of this chapter, the reader will be able to:

- describe and critique the division of labour in rural communities

- discuss and critique employment opportunities in rural Australia

- debate the impact of the mining boom on rural Australia

- outline the major healthcare issues of working adults in rural Australia

- explain the role and function of the nurse in providing health care to adults in rural communities.

Key words Adults, rural, employment, division of labour, nurses

Chapter overview

The adult in rural settings is the focus of this chapter. In it we will discuss how employment openings present themselves as opportunities for adults to settle and grow in rural areas. According to Reimer (1997), informal social networks assist with gaining employment or developing employment opportunities in rural areas. Changes in kin and friendship relationships, divisions of labour and economic viability also impinge on rural employment. When economic factors threaten the viability of local employers, unemployment challenges arise – and these will also be discussed. Common health conditions and serious threats to wellbeing from either those employed or those not employed will be outlined. The central role of nurses in various practice settings and their interaction with the adult population will be weaved through the discussions.

Gender and work

More than one-third of Australians live in rural and regional areas (see Chapters 1 and 2). However, many rural areas are characterised by an ageing and declining population. Young people and families migrate to urban centres for improved work, education and lifestyle opportunities. Gender equality within rural areas enables women to become viable economic players in sustaining employment. Gender norms and patterns can be rigid in some countries; women are often placed in a disadvantaged position to men. Unequal pay, hours of employment and rights of the individual are all factors that contribute to such inequality (Food and Agricultural Organization of the United Nations [FAO], 2010). When women are equal contributing partners in a household, the health of that household increases, and women's leadership and decision-making participation are also strengthened (FAO, 2010). The Australian Bureau of Statistics (ABS) (2006) reported that, in 2001, participation in the labour force for women was 65.3% compared to men at 80.4%. Small towns had the highest proportion of female part-time workers at 54.3% compared to rural areas at 51.9%.

Rural employment includes farming, self-employment, trades and professions, and small enterprises providing goods and services. Some of this work done by women involves long hours and is not sufficiently remunerated. In Australian rural society, the superiority of men and the inferiority of women exist. Men control the most valued resources – farming land, town businesses and executive positions. They also dominate political, community services and recreational activities and delegate domestic tasks and child care to women. Women also constitute a significant proportion of unpaid family workers; they care for the sick or injured and help on the family farm by performing unpaid hard labour or managing the business books. These unpaid hours often go unnoticed by society, yet government savings because of this unrecognised work are significant and constitute substantial savings to the public purse.

ACTIVITY

Look at the structure and function of the following organisations in a rural community with which you are familiar.
> Local government (council)
> Chamber of Commerce
> Museum
> Library
> University
> Hospital and health care
> Bank
> Supermarket
> Greengrocery store
> Local transport system (bus or coach).
   ● How many men versus women serve within the organisation?
   ● What are the roles of men versus women in the organisation?
   ● How many organisations have a woman holding an executive position?

You may find that, in most organisations, it is men who hold the positions of influence and women who are subordinate. Perhaps this is so in all of the organisations except health and health care, where women dominate. However, in line with the national average, men in health care seem to rise to the top quickly and usually by exploitation of women. What did you find?

Employment opportunities

Attracting and retaining people to work in rural areas are sometimes extremely difficult. Health agencies – and primarily those employing doctors – offer attractive packages that include accommodation and salary increases to overcome such shortages of qualified personnel. Despite these incentives, it is significantly difficult to attract and retain doctors in rural areas. There are no such incentives to encourage nurses to rural areas, yet there is a constant shortage of nursing personnel.

A study into rural employment called for a coordinating role within rural areas to avoid duplication of efforts, competition within regions and better efficiency. 'The group could consist of representatives from major employment sectors, local business groups, training providers and relevant government agencies' (Rural Industries Research and Development Corporation [RIRDC], 2009, p. xv). The study also proposed that finding quality accommodation and subsidising living costs were also an attractive lure for those seeking jobs. Provision of adequate and relevant social and lifestyle recreational facilities is often missing from rural towns and thus is a disincentive for people to settle into these communities.

Professionals who move between rural towns are more likely to remain if their social and professional needs are met. Skilled newcomers seeking a sea change or lifestyle change are often driven by the possibility of a safe haven to bring up children or the development of new professional opportunities (Kilpatrick, Johns, Vitartas & Homisan, 2011). Partner satisfaction rates are a key to the recruitment and retention of skilled workers in rural areas (Han & Humphreys, 2005). Skilled newcomers and their families' transition into rural populations can take time, and small rural communities are not always welcoming (Smailes, 2002). Community identity may be threatened or divided (Gray & Sinclair, 2005). Newcomers have to demonstrate that they have the capacity to strengthen the community's social capital. Communities have a key role in the integration process and they need to ease in the newcomers, matching their social needs with what the community can offer (Kilpatrick et al., 2011).

Let's take a closer look at employment opportunities that are common to rural areas.

Farming

Agriculture has been named the driver of rural employment. Yet rural family farming appears to be on the decline with the need to constantly modernise machinery (Stayner, 2005). These new technologies are often costly and beyond the small farmer's budget, and the cost-price squeeze has forced large numbers of farmers from the land and made way for more profitable producers to expand their operations (RIRDC, 2009). Economic pressures are not the only issue facing farmers; climate change has seriously affected agricultural production. Drought, rising salinity and resultant poor soils cement the widely held perception that careers in agriculture are limited and farmers face seemingly never-ending problems (House of Representatives Standing Committee on Agriculture, Fisheries and Forestry, 2007). The former Australian Greenhouse Office's guide to climate science and impacts records some of the outcomes of climate change:

- a decrease in available water resources
- higher temperatures and hence evaporation
- increased heat stress of livestock causing reduced weight and milk yields
- reduction in chilling cultivars, viticulture yields
- damage of crops from extreme weather, increased pests and disease outbreaks
- a reduction of area of arable land from the 'dustbowl effect', and
- a reduction of crop yield and quality (Climate Action Network Australia, 2013).

In short, a career in agriculture seems only viable for large farming consortia and those able to afford the technology to keep it going (see Chapter 2). There are exceptions, however; the case study of Oberon warrants further explanation.

VIGNETTE

Oberon is situated in the Blue Mountains in New South Wales. It is approximately 196 km west of Sydney and lies 1113 metres above sea level. It has extremes of climate, from snow to extreme heat. Traditionally, Oberon boasts 150 years of family farming – livestock, crops and agriculture. The agricultural industry declined as a result of increased costs, low exports and competing imports. In 1996 the population was 2600, of which 87.4% were Australian born of English or Anglo-Saxon origin. The average weekly household income was $623 (compared with the Australian average of $635).

》》 The effect of world trading patterns for wool led to a decline in the wool industry in Oberon. Sheep farms became unprofitable. However, the strength of the people in Oberon lies in their ability to diversify. Oberon made a successful change from primary industry (beef cattle and lamb) to pine trees as a secondary industry with input from large companies such as Boral and CSR. Almost 50% of the surrounding area is state forest and radiated pine tree plantations. Alongside this development there is a growing small agricultural crop development – vegetables, trees and bulbs. Tourism has developed, with the small surrounding historic villages offering farm stays, chalets and cabins, bed and breakfast, hotels, motels and caravan parks. All this is within easy reach of Sydney's urban sprawl.

Farmers in Oberon have used their initiative and teamed together to become progressive. They have been able to maintain some traditional farming practices whilst using the land in other ways to make money. Hobby farming has grown within the area, where older, larger farms have been subdivided to make smaller, more manageable lots; this is despite them being categorised as some of the most difficult lands to farm. This diversification of land by former farmers has created a new employment status – that of rural managers.

The pine tree development led to a softwood industry, and a sawmill emerged. With input from CSR and Boral, the sawmill employs 150 local people to man this operation 24/7. This sawmill development also manufactures mulch from the timber processing and thus feeds into the local landscaping businesses.

In short, the Oberon community has accepted the cultural and industrial changes, yet it holds onto the natural heritage and has adapted to survive.

Fly-in, fly-out/drive-in, drive-out

In recent years, mining has played a crucial role in regional Australia. It is a major generator of earnings and jobs. Driven by demand from Asia, namely China and Japan, expansion has occurred in a wide range of commodities including iron ore, bauxite, nickel, gold, mineral sands, oil, gas and coal. Mining has also realised demands in supporting occupations such as geoscience and construction. Mining is widely dispersed across rural and regional Australia, and attracting employees in the current era of rapid growth in relatively remote locations has led to the expansion of the 'fly-in, fly-out/drive-in, drive-out' (FIFO/DIDO) labour force. FIFO is not new to the Australian mining industry. Indeed, FIFO practices were established as early as 1960. Of late, however, FIFO has expanded because of supply and demand increases and new mines being established in rural or remote Australia. Employees of these mines can be from the local areas, but more often they come from interstate metropolitan cities or large regional towns and fly or drive to the mines for their rostered shifts, which can be anything from five days on and five days off to three weeks on and three weeks off. High wages, provision of living quarters, food and leisure activities, cars and good working conditions attract men and women who are prepared to leave their families behind in metropolitan cities or larger regional centres.

The workforce is largely full-time, with 97% of workers engaged in full-time employment. The workforce attracts an older person, and the median age of workers is 40 years compared with 37 years for the national workforce (House of Representatives Standing Committee on Regional Australia, 2013). There is a paucity of information regarding the actual FIFO presence in the resource industry. A survey conducted by the Chamber of Commerce and Industry Western Australia in 2005 attempted to glean some data regarding FIFO workers. They claimed:

- 76.5% of all personnel were employed directly by mining companies
- 23.5% of all personnel were employed by contractors
- 53% of all mining employees (contractors and direct employees) were employed on a residential basis
- 47% of all mining employees were employed on a FIFO basis, including 4.7% utilising DIDO arrangements
- 62.5% of directly employed personnel are residential and 37.5% are FIFO, and
- 22.3% of contractor personnel are residential and 77.7% are FIFO (House of Representatives Standing Committee on Regional Australia, 2013, p. 16).

The Committee reported that the lack of comprehensive nationwide data was problematic, and the lack of data and its effects on planning, funding and the formulation of policy was a major finding of the report. As the mining boom grew, Australia became the world's largest economic resource of brown coal, mineral sands, nickel, silver, uranium, zinc and lead and attracted multinational resource companies to invest in Australia's natural wealth.

However, FIFO work is not without its risks. The House of Representatives' inquiry (2013) into FIFO work arrangements allowed many anecdotal submissions. Numbers of people remarked that they disliked aspects of the workplace and lifestyle intensely but felt trapped because they had high financial commitments based on their high salaries, compounded by the lack of viable employment opportunities in their home cities (Hoath & McKenzie, 2013). Other anecdotes revealed that some workers missed out on birthday celebrations within their families and holidays such as Easter and Christmas. If relationships became difficult, then there were mental health issues, substance abuse and even suicides (Hoath & McKenzie, 2013). However, Griffith University's Australian Institute for Suicide Research and Prevention refutes the claim of more suicides among miners, suggesting that their study claimed there was a lot of myth-making about the life of a FIFO/DIDO worker and that mental health matters were exaggerated for effect (as cited in McPhedran, 2013). Nevertheless, their study did claim that miners experienced stress, anxiety, divorce, drug and alcohol usage and a sense of helplessness (Santhebennur, 2013).

Spouses of FIFO/DIDO workers reported that being part of a FIFO family tended to place them in a situation where local businesses would charge extra for service. When the worker comes home, they experience local charities asking them for money because they earn a high income. One worker said that he was doing this work to bolster his superannuation and looked forward to a comfortable retirement.

Issues of high rents were also brought to the House of Representatives Committee. One claim showed that rents in a rural and isolated town reached as high as $1500/week. These prices suit the mining companies that place six or more men in a house, but normal families cannot pay these exorbitant amounts. In his submission to the Committee, Professor Drew Dawson from Central Queensland University suggested that mining companies take more responsibility by conducting social impact assessments of each mining area (ABC News, 2013).

Access to healthcare services is a well-recognised problem for people living in rural areas. Sudden population growth as a result of the expansion of FIFO/DIDO workers can exert pressures on local infrastructure and service capability, thus worsening access to these vital facilities (McPhedran, 2013). Professor Kerry Carrington from Queensland's University of Technology has conducted a wide-ranging study of the social impacts of mining and is mindful of the health impacts FIFO workers bring upon themselves. She claims that the mining living arrangements could be likened to a holiday camp and that when workers become bored during the extended periods of work, they engage in risky behaviours such as drinking excessively, taking illicit drugs and engaging in sexual experimentation (Safety WA, 2011). Carrington (Safety WA, 2011) warns that regular check-ups as part of normal family life are often ignored, and tooth decay and eye deterioration become major problems for this group of individuals.

Manufacturing

Since the liberalisation of the economy in the 1970s, international competition has threatened manufacturing in regional Australia. High local wages, taxes and stringent environmental regulations have resulted in a large number of firms collapsing or taking their businesses offshore (O'Connor, Stimson & Daly, 2001). In spite of this turmoil, manufacturing still features as a vital element of the economies of regional areas. RIRDC (2009) suggests that two areas that are valued are 'mineral processing and food and beverage production' (p. 7). Western Australia and Queensland harness mineral processing, while South Australia, Western Australia, New South Wales and Victoria have a high number of large-scale industries in food and beverage, including wine production. Linked in part to tourism and lifestyle migration, smaller 'boutique' style enterprises have experienced resurgence. However, Tonts, Davies and Haslam-McKenzie (2008) note that there is much anecdotal evidence to suggest that a number of these small enterprises have experienced problems in attracting and retaining labour as a result of strong competition from mining companies offering higher wages.

Education hubs

Education in rural Australia has come to the fore in recent years. Driven by several forces such as the value of the economic and social contributions made by country people and country communities, the rapidly expanding internet and technologies mean that several rural and regional centres are home to universities in their own right or campuses of metropolitan universities. As such, these organisations provide employment at several levels. Some universities have joined forces with technical and further education organisations (and trade training centres) and schools, and they have become a hub for easy transition from one organisation to another (e.g. Federation University at Gippsland and Ballarat, and Central Queensland University at Mackay, Rockhampton and Bundaberg). With positive discrimination and engagement on their agenda, these organisations also become centres for employment for Aboriginal and Torres Strait Islander people of Australia.

Indigenous Youth Careers Pathways Program was an initiative of the Labor government in 2011–2012. It provided funds to a school-based traineeship to assist Indigenous young men and women to have a seamless pathway from school to further vocational training, education or a job. Centred in areas of low socioeconomic status with viable labour markets, this incentive was geared towards regional and rural centres or larger cities rather than remote areas (a different funding scheme exists in remote areas). The other strategy that is directed towards Aboriginal and Torres Strait Islander people is the Indigenous Employment Program (IEP), which offers funding for activities focused on employment, training, aspiration building and business support. The IEP funds projects that:

- encourage and support employers to provide sustainable employment opportunities
- encourage and support Indigenous Australians to take up training and employment opportunities, stay in jobs and enhance their future employment prospects
- develop the Indigenous workforce and economic development strategies that support local and regional economic growth, and
- develop sustainable Indigenous businesses and economic opportunities in urban, regional and remote areas (Australian Government Budget, 2012–13).

Education hubs attract highly qualified professors and academics, but they would not function without a host of support personnel. Administrative staff, maintenance staff, builders, mechanics, gardeners and cleaners all help keep these large organisations viable. Government funding of over $19.1 million to 2014 was granted to employ 34 regional education, skills and job coordinators to work in regional communities across the country:

> These coordinators work with community stakeholders, including Regional Development Australia Committees, to develop Regional Education, Skills and Jobs Plans that include strategies to improve participation and outcomes in education, training and employment in regional Australia. The Regional Education, Skills and Jobs Coordinators are working to ensure communities are aware of the opportunities available including facilitating linkages across Government programs (Australian Government Budget, 2012–13).

It is likely that these coordinators will provide a more engaged compilation of job and learning opportunities for people in rural areas.

Gaols and forensics

Building prisons in rural areas delivers substantial fiscal increases to rural towns because they are a recession-proof form of monetary expansion (Whitfield, 2008; Besser & Hanson, 2004). This positive feature, however, is offset with a number of challenges such as accommodating socioeconomic, educational and recreational needs of itinerant populations that relocate to be close to incarcerated relatives (Milne, 2013). Gaol towns are often stigmatised because people fear the impact on personal safety, property values and overall quality of life (Besser & Hanson, 2004).

Unemployment

Gaining accurate and up-to-date figures on the level of rural unemployment is almost impossible. In 1966, the total unemployment rate in Australian rural areas was 6.7% compared to 8.2% in towns and 6.6% in urban areas. The ABS data go back to the late 1990s or early to mid 2000s. Areas of high unemployment as described by the ABS are captured in Table 7.1.

TABLE 7.1 *Statistical Local Areas (SLA) in each state/territory with the highest unemployment figures.*

STATE/TERRITORY	SUBDIVISION	UNEMPLOYMENT (%)	LABOUR FORCE PARTICIPATION (%)	MEDIAN AGE (YEARS)
NSW	Clarence (excl. Coffs Harbour)	15.0	50.0	41
VIC	La Trobe Valley	12.0	59.0	35
QLD	Hervey Bay City Part A	14.9	43.9	43
SA	Whyalla	13.2	57.8	35
WA	Mandurah	12.4	53.0	39
TAS	Burnie–Devonport	12.5	55.7	37
NT	Bathurst–Melville	13.1	47.1	24
ACT	North Canberra	6.9	66.5	32

(Adapted from ABS, 2001, Census of Population and Housing, as cited in *Australian Social Trends*, ABS, 2003)

Unemployment rates range widely across SLAs. While there is variation across states, there is also a tendency for adjoining SLAs within a state or territory to share similar trends for unemployment (ABS, 2003). For example, the long coastal belt of northern NSW and southern Queensland had an unemployment rate of 10% (ABS, 2003). Men in rural areas have slightly higher rates of unemployment than women.

The labour force for women in rural Australia is interesting. The ABS reports that women in rural areas are least likely to be unemployed and most likely to be self-employed, with at least half of them working in agriculture (ABS, 2006). The proportion of unemployed people who were Indigenous rose with increasing remoteness. In 2001, Aboriginal and Torres Strait Islander people made up a greater proportion of unemployed people in very remote areas (42%), remote areas (21.3%), outer regional areas (9%), inner regional areas (4%)

and major cities (2%). At each level of remoteness, the Indigenous unemployment rate was three times higher than the non-Indigenous rate (ABS, 2003).

The most up-to-date figure for unemployment nationally is 5.7% of the working population (Australian Government, 2013). Unemployment can be short term or long term. People who are unemployed for more than one year are categorised as being long-term unemployed. Many who have been out of work for a long time experience a loss of confidence and motivation for finding work. Some may even experience negative perceptions of potential employers because they have been unemployed for so long. Table 7.2 denotes the areas that had relatively high rates of long-term unemployment in 2001.

TABLE 7.2 *Areas with relatively high rates of long-term unemployment in 2001.*

STATISTICAL REGION OR SECTOR/S	%
Hunter (a) – NSW	3.7
Mersey–Lyell (b) – TAS	3.5
North Western Melbourne (a) – VIC	3.4
Wide Bay–Burnett (a) – QLD	3.4
Northern and Western SA (a) – SA	3.1
Greater Hobart–Southern (b) – TAS	3.1
Northern Adelaide (a) – SA	2.8
Northern (b) – TAS	2.7
Gold Coast City Parts A and B (c) – QLD	2.7
Loddon–Mallee (a) – VIC	2.7
Western Adelaide (a) – SA	2.5

(Adapted from ABS, 2003)

Unemployment does not just affect the person without a job; family members and the wider community can also be affected. Unemployment is also a loss of productive resources to the economy and at a personal level often affects living standards into retirement. Work is strongly linked to identity, and if unemployment occurs at a mature age it can create family tensions or self-abuse, violence or crime.

Government monetary incentives are muted for 18–30-year-olds to find work and stay employed, with the person who is long-term unemployed to receive $2500 when they start a position and stay off welfare for 12 months. An additional $400 will be paid if they stay in work and remain off welfare (Walsh, 2013). However, many young people choose not to work full-time so will not be able to receive these incentives. Generation X value their leisure time and are not motivated to work 36 hours/week or more.

There will always be unemployment. For the most part it is a state of transiency, and those unemployed in one week will find suitable work positions in the next week. Nevertheless, the fallout from unemployment can bring with it mental health issues, and rural nurses should be well versed in recognising the signs of low self-esteem, depression and potential suicide.

Nurses' roles in supporting the adult population

Nurses who work in rural areas are often part of the community in which they practise. Mills, Francis and Bonner (2007) suggest that, because of their attachment to the community, they actually live their work. They can become compromised at times because they often personally know their patients. Yet they also have an overwhelming concern for the community in which they live and work and the quality of the service they can provide (Mills et al., 2007). They also value their colleagues and engage in mentoring their subordinates to provide the same quality care (Mills et al., 2007). Rural nurses have to maintain a wide skills range to cater for the diverse needs of people in their community and must often 'make do' with inadequate tools or materials. Rural nurses must also present multiple faces to the community: the caring nurse, the advocate, the negotiator, the mentor, the teacher, the politician.

Screening women and men

Establishing respectful partnerships between communities and individuals is one of the cornerstone processes of good primary health care. It is person-centred and incorporates a holistic approach of the body, mind, spirit, land, environment, culture and custom (Adrian, 2009).

Women are taught at an early age to test for breast lumps and have regular Pap smears if they are sexually active. In the main, Australian women are reasonably committed to attend to these two major health issues. Nevertheless, the rural nurse must be mindful of the social determinants of health and acknowledge that not all women are equipped with the knowledge to follow through with these procedures. Rural nurses may be invited to talk about these screening tools at schools, universities or workplaces, and they have to be skilled in making presentations to public audiences.

Men have become more proactive about their health, and as such this self-care has increased men's life expectancy rates in Australia. It could also be argued that health education and awareness of what to do if certain symptoms appear have contributed to raising awareness of ill-health. Denner (2003) argues that men need to feel they have some knowledge before they will attend a general practitioner (GP) for assistance – they need to feel in control. Thus it is important for rural nurses to stay up to date with the latest protocols on such treatments as cardiopulmonary resuscitation. The other intervention that can be lifesaving is a check for prostate cancer. Conducting men's health groups for men of all ages could assist in getting recalcitrant males to seek assistance from their GP.

Common health complaints and interventions

Rural Australian adults experience the spectrum of chronic diseases such as diabetes, heart disease, arthritis and asthma, as do other Australian adults (Australian Institute of Health and Welfare [AIHW], 2008). Health outcomes for Aboriginal and Torres Strait Islander rural adults are acknowledged as being worse than for non-Indigenous rural adults, despite affirmative actions by all levels of government (Australian Human Rights Commission, 2012).

The perversity of living in rural settings means access to health care and other supports are limited, thus increasing the burden of disease on individuals and communities (AIHW, 2008). The incidence of cancers in the rural adult population is slightly higher than for metropolitan populations and is significantly higher for preventable cancers such as melanoma, lung, head and neck, and lip cancers than those of the broader Australian population (AIHW, 2008; Phillips, 2009). Mental health disorders are a leading cause of disease burden and injury, with anxiety, depression, alcohol abuse and personality disorders the most common (AIHW, 2008; Phillips, 2009). Rural male suicide rates are higher than for non-rural populations and are significantly influenced by the number of suicides of young Aboriginal and Torres Strait Islander men living in very remote settings (Phillips, 2009). Poor oral health has been highlighted as a feature of the rural populations' health status, particularly for Aboriginal and Torres Strait Islander populations (Phillips, 2009). Behaviours, lower levels of income and education, poorer infrastructure and increased occupational and environmental health risks are recognised as risk factors that contribute to the burden of disease and injury experienced by rural adults (Phillips, 2009).

Trauma, triage and evacuation

Injury is a leading cause of death among Australians aged 1–44 years and the fifth leading cause of hospitalisation for all ages (Mitchell & Chong, 2010). Rural people have an increased likelihood of being injured and/or dying from workplace injury, motor vehicle accidents, interpersonal violence, suicide and self-inflicted wounds, electrocution, drowning, falls and poisoning (AIHW, 2008; Mitchell & Chong, 2010). Rural males are at higher risk than rural females, although both genders are more susceptible to fatal and non-fatal injury than their large city counterparts (Mitchell & Chong, 2010). Furthermore, morbidity and mortality associated with motor vehicle accidents in rural and remote Australia are double those of capital cities (McDonell, Veitch, Aitken & Elcock, 2009).

Trauma resulting from injury has been the impetus for growth in pre-emergency and disaster management health care that is inclusive of point-of-injury triage, stabilisation and evacuation. In rural contexts especially, time is a crucial factor in managing injury that is potentially life-threatening, irrespective of causation (Tazarourte et al., 2013). Triage involves a systematic method for rating injury according to the level of urgency, and the corresponding actions that include where to evacuate to are required to sustain life while minimising preventable disability (Kennedy, Aghababian, Gans & Lewis, 1996). Stabilising the injured involves treating immediate threats to life such as blood loss, head and neck injury, fractures, cardiac output and airway compromise. Retrieval involves the physical removal of the stabilised injured to a transport vehicle such as an ambulance or aircraft for transfer to a hospital (Lockey & Deakin, 2005; Wong & Petchell, 2004). Pre-emergency healthcare teams include paramedics, nurses and doctors.

VIGNETTE

Peter, aged 60, and his wife Dianne, aged 56, are on a caravan trip around the 'top end' (north) of Australia. Peter has hypertension and diabetes and is overweight. He has an extensive list of medications to manage the hypertension and is on insulin to manage his mature age onset diabetes. Dianne is being treated for hypertension and asthma. She is also overweight. Neither of them engages in regular exercise. Both consider themselves to be 'average' drinkers, consuming about three standard drinks (beer for Peter and wine for Dianne) per day. Peter is the main driver. Dianne does drive occasionally but is unable to reverse park the caravan, change tyres or attend to any routine maintenance.

⟩⟩ About 30 minutes out of a small rural town, Peter starts to slur his speech and says he feels 'funny'. Dianne takes over the driving and, by the time they arrive in the town, Peter has had a stroke. Dianne finds the hospital and a nurse comes from the wards into the emergency area. She assesses Peter and telephones the doctor who practises in the town. The doctor attends, provides emergency treatment and organises for Peter to be sent to the regional centre by plane. The whole process takes about four hours. Dianne is unable to accompany her husband on the retrieval aircraft and is left to find the caravan park and park the caravan. She manages to do this with the assistance of other caravan owners and the owner of the caravan park. Dianne calls her children to let them know what is happening. They live in another state and are at least two plane flights away from where she is. Dianne is now about five hours' drive from the hospital where her husband has been sent. There is a domestic airline, so she organises to fly on that to her husband. As she is about to leave, she is advised that her husband has not survived.

Dianne is now left in a strange town, with a car and caravan that she is unable to drive. She has to leave both and fly to where her husband has died in order to make arrangements for his remains to be sent back to their hometown (after the autopsy). Dianne is aware that she needs to organise the funeral and address her family's immediate spiritual and emotional needs. She also requires someone to fly to the town, retrieve the car and caravan and get them back to her place of abode.

While this sounds dramatic, it is not unusual and is a good demonstration of the isolation of rural communities and the limited capacity of small health services to cope with growing numbers of visitors.

Summary

In this chapter, we have covered:

- factors impacting on gender roles and opportunities for employment in rural areas
- common areas of employment in rural areas
- the impact of unemployment for adults in rural areas
- the role of the nurse supporting rural adults
- common health complaints in rural Australia.

Reflective questions

1 Think about the role of women in rural society – what are their employment opportunities and, if not gainfully employed, how do they contribute to the fabric of rural communities?

2 What opportunities are open to young people in rural communities who are just leaving school? Are they advantaged/disadvantaged in any way compared to their urban counterparts?

3   What impact on local communities does a mining boom offer?
4   If you were gainfully employed in agriculture in a rural area, what might be your health risks?
5   As a nurse in a rural town, what might be your scope of practice?

References

ABC News. (2013, February 14). FIFO report offers 'balanced' view. Retrieved December 4, 2013, from http://www.abc.net.au/news/2013–02–14/fifo-report-offers-balanced-view/4518282

Adrian, A. (2009). *Primary health care in Australia: A nursing and midwifery consensus view*. Rozelle, NSW: Australian Nurses Federation.

Australian Bureau of Statistics (ABS). (2003). *4102.0 – Australian Social Trends, 2003*. Canberra: Australian Government. Retrieved December 5, 2013, from http://www.abs.gov.au/AUSSTATS/abs@.nsf/2f762f95845417aeca25706c00834efa/479960b75bb5469eca2570ec00006ee8!OpenDocument

——. (2006). *Perspectives on regional Australia: Women's employment in urban, rural and regional Australia, 2001 Census*. Canberra: Australian Government. Retrieved December 5, 2013, from http://www.abs.gov.au/AUSSTATS/abs@.nsf/Lookup/1380.0.55.001Main+Features12001

Australian Government. (2013). Labour force region. Department of Employment. Retrieved December 5, 2013, from http://lmip.gov.au/default.aspx?LMIP/LFR

Australian Government Budget. (2012–13). Education, employment and workplace relations. Retrieved December 5, 2013, from http://www.budget.gov.au/2012-13/content/ministerial_statements/rural_and_regional/html/rural_and_regional-08.htm

Australian Human Rights Commission. (2012). Close the gap: Indigenous health campaign. Retrieved December 9, 2013, from http://www.humanrights.gov.au/close-gap-indigenous-health-campaign

Australian Institute of Health and Welfare (AIHW). (2008). *Rural, regional and remote health: Indicators of health status and determinants of health*. Canberra: Australian Government. Retrieved December 9, 2013, from http://www.aihw.gov.au/WorkArea/DownloadAsset.aspx?id=6442459831

Besser, T. L. & Hanson, M. M. (2004). Focus on rural economic development. *Journal of the Community Development Society*, 35(2), 1–16. doi: 10.1080/15575330409490129

Climate Action Network Australia. (2013). Social impacts of climate change: Farming and rural communities. Retrieved December 5, 2013, from http://www.cana.net.au/socialimpacts/index.html

Denner, B. (2003, March). National men's health policy. Paper presented at the 7th National Rural Health Conference, Hobart, Tasmania.

Food and Agricultural Organization of the United Nations (FAO). (2010). *Gender dimensions of agricultural and rural employment: Differentiated pathways out of poverty*. Rome: FAO, the International Fund for Agricultural Development and the International Labour Office. Retrieved March 24, 2014, from http://www.fao.org/docrep/013/i1638e/i1638e.pdf

Gray, I. & Sinclair, P. (2005). Local leaders in a global setting: Dependency and resistance in regional New South Wales and Newfoundland. *Sociologia Ruralis*, 45(1–2), 37–52. doi: 10.1111/j.1467–9523.2005.00289.x

Han, G. S. & Humphreys, J. S. (2005). Overseas-trained doctors in Australia: Community integration and their intention to stay in a rural community. *Australian Journal of Rural Health*, 13(4), 236–41. doi: 10.1111/j.1440–1584.2005.00708.x

Hoath, A. & McKenzie, F. (2013, November 25). Fly-in fly-out worth the pain, for some: Study. *Australian Mining*. Retrieved December 4, 2013, from http://www.miningaustralia.com.au/features/fly-in-fly-out-worth-the-pain-for-some-study

House of Representatives Standing Committee on Agriculture, Fisheries and Forestry. (2007). *Skills: Rural Australia's need: Inquiry into rural skills training and research*. Canberra: Commonwealth of Australia. Retrieved March 24, 2014, from http://www.daff.gov.au/__data/assets/pdf_file/0013/1530022/govt-resphor-rural_skills.pdf

House of Representatives Standing Committee on Regional Australia. (2013). *Cancer of the bush or salvation for our cities? Fly-in, fly-out and drive-in, drive-out workforce practices in regional Australia*. Canberra: Commonwealth of Australia. Retrieved March 24, 2014, from http://www.aph.gov.au/parliamentary_business/committees/house_of_representatives_committees?url=ra/fifodido/report.htm

Kennedy, K., Aghababian, R. V., Gans, L. & Lewis, C. P. (1996). Triage: Techniques and applications in decision making. *Annals of Emergency Medicine*, 28(2), 136–44. doi: http://dx.doi.org/10.1016/S0196-0644(96)70053-7

Kilpatrick, S., Johns, S., Vitartas, P. & Homisan, M. (2011). Mobile skilled workers: Making the most of an untapped rural community resource. *Journal of Rural Studies*, 27(2), 181–90. http://dx.doi.org/10.1016/j.jrurstud.2011.01.003

Lockey, D. & Deakin, C. D. (2005). Pre-hospital trauma care: Systems and delivery. *Continuing Education in Anaesthesia, Critical Care & Pain*, 5(6), 191–4. doi: 10.1093/bjaceaccp/mki054

McDonell, A. C., Veitch, C., Aitken, P. & Elcock, M. (2009). The organisation of trauma services for rural Australia. *Journal of Emergency Primary Health Care*, 7(2).

McPhedran, S. (2013, January 17). Mining, fly-in, fly-out workers and the risk of suicide. *Australian Mining*. Retrieved December 4, 2013, from http://www.miningaustralia.com.au/features/mining-fly-in-fly-out-workers-and-the-risk-of-suic

Mills, J., Francis, K. & Bonner, A. (2007). Live my work: Rural nurses and their multiple perspectives of self. *Journal of Advanced Nursing*, 59(6), 583–90. doi: 10.1111/j.1365–2648.2007.04350.x

Milne, S. (2013). Grafton community fuming over 'heartless' goal downsizing. *Green Left Weekly*. Retrieved December 9, 2013, from http://www.greenleft.org.au/node/51615

Mitchell, R. J. & Chong, S. (2010). Comparison of injury-related hospitalised morbidity and mortality in urban and rural areas in Australia. *Rural and Remote Health*, 10(1326), 1–10. Retrieved March 24, 2014, from http://www.rrh.org.au/publishedarticles/article_print_1326.pdf

O'Connor, K., Stimson, R. & Daly, M. (2001). *Australia's changing economic geography*. Melbourne: Oxford University Press.

Phillips, A. (2009). Health status differentials across rural and remote Australia. *Australian Journal of Rural Health*, 17(1), 2–9. doi: 10.1111/j.1440-1584.2008.01029.x

Reimer, B. (1997). Informal rural networks: Their contribution to 'making a living' and creating rural employment. In R. D. Bollman & J. M. Bryden (Eds.), *Rural employment: An international perspective* (pp. 396–409). Oxon, UK: CAB International.

Rural Industries Research and Development Corporation (RIRDC). (2009). *Australia's rural workforce: An analysis of labour shortages in rural Australia*. Canberra: Commonwealth of Australia. Retrieved March 24, 2014, from https://rirdc.infoservices.com.au/items/09-008

Safety WA. (2011, December). Many submissions to FIFO inquiry. *West Australian Journal of Occupational Safety and Health*. Retrieved December 4, 2013, from http://www.ifap.asn.au/Documents/Publications/SafetyWA%202011/safetywadecember_2011_web%20%282%29.pdf

Santhebennur, M. (2013, August 6). Male miners' mental health claims overblown: Research. *Australian Mining*. Retrieved December, 4, 2013, from http://www.miningaustralia.com.au/news/male-miners-mental-health-claims-overblown-researc

Smailes, P. J. (2002). From rural dilution to multifunctional countryside: Some pointers to the future from South Australia. *Australian Geographer*, 33(1), 79–95.

Stayner, R. (2005). The changing economics of rural communities. In C. Cocklin & J. Dibdin (Eds.), *Sustainability and change in rural Australia* (pp. 129–409). Sydney: University of NSW Press.

Tazarourte, K., Cesaréo, E., Sapir, D., Atchabahian, A., Tourtier, J. P., Briole, N. & Vigué, B. (2013). Update on prehospital emergency care of severe trauma patients. *Annales Françaises d'Anesthésie et de Réanimation*, 32(7/8), 477–82. doi: 10.1016/j.annfar.2013.07.005

Tonts, M., Davies, A. & Haslam-McKenzie, F. (2008). *Regional workforce futures: An analysis of the great southern, south west and wheatbelt regions*. Geowest No 35, Institute for Regional Development. Perth: The University of Western Australia. Retrieved March 24, 2014, from http://espace.library.curtin.edu.au/cgi-bin/espace.pdf?file=/2009/03/16/file_1/118029

Walsh, L. (2013). Incentives not enough to tackle youth unemployment. The Drum Opinion, ABC. Retrieved December 5, 2013, from http://www.abc.net.au/news/2013-08-28/walsh-incentives-not-enough-to-tackle-youth-unemployment/4919112

Whitfield, D. (2008). *Economic impact of prisons in rural areas*. Adelaide: European Services Strategy Unit. Retrieved March 24, 2014, from http://www.european-services-strategy.org.uk/outsourcing-library/pfi-ppp/economic-impact-of-prisons-in-rural-areas-a-re/prison-impact-review.doc

Wong, K. & Petchell, J. (2004). Resources for managing trauma in rural New South Wales, Australia. *ANZ Journal of Surgery*, 74(9), 760–5. doi: 10.1111/j.1445-1433.2004.03138.x

8 Living longer, living well

Judith Anderson, Carmel Davies and Mary FitzGerald

Learning objectives

On completion of this chapter, the reader will be able to:

- empathise with older people in rural Australian communities

- discuss the attitudes towards healthy ageing in rural communities and their association with living well

- identify the role that lay carers play in support for older people with healthcare needs

- identify the role that professional health services play in the maintenance of healthy lifestyles for older people in rural communities

- appreciate the advantages for older people, their carers and family members of preparing advanced care directives.

Key words

- Living well, chronic and complex care, self-care, health promotion, advanced care directives

Chapter overview

This chapter provides a positive picture of living well as an older person in a rural community. It covers self-care and formal and informal support services for older people by profiling a fictional senior Australian, Sarah Atwood, as she becomes frail and in need of extra support.

Introduction

Community is a key word in rural living as it signals benefits of mateship, reciprocity and security. These are particularly valued aspects of rural living for older people and can make the difference between a contented old age and one full of ill-health, social isolation and insecurity. Active older people are the backbone of any rural community through the contribution of their time and talents to family life as informal and formal carers for partners, friends and family. They also get involved in politics, voluntary services, social networks and charities. Such activities keep people interested and involved and add substantially to feelings of self-worth and dignity, which are so necessary for mental health and wellbeing.

In this chapter there is a focus on healthy living for older people, with particular reference to living in a rural community. While a great deal has been written about the disparities between health services in urban and rural Australia, it will be argued that there is a need to concentrate on living well and creating an atmosphere where old age is viewed by all in the community – especially young people – as a stage in life that has as much potential for happiness as any other stage. To illustrate this, snapshots are provided of the life of Sarah Atwood, a fictional senior Australian living in a rural community, as she gradually ages and becomes frail.

Rural people are renowned for their resilience and independence, and therefore Orem's self-care agency will be used to explain levels of intervention required with older people. According to Orem, the self-care agent is the person who provides for any person's universal self-care needs: air, water, nutrition, elimination, balance between rest and activity, balance between solitude and social interaction, and safety and society (as cited in Pearson, Vaughan & FitzGerald, 2005). In good health a person acts as their own self-care agent, balancing demands with their ability to meet them; at this stage, nursing offers a supportive educative service. When the balance between ability and demand is disturbed by ill-health or loss of function, a partially compensatory system is adopted where support is provided by other agents such as family and friends or health professionals. As the goal is self-care, any improvement in ability is accompanied by a gradual reduction in compensatory care.

The next sections will follow Orem's systems of care, beginning with supportive educative care of older people in rural communities who are most likely to be as healthy as the majority of other people in the community. It is a seldom acknowledged fact, when considering the 'problem' associated with the ageing of Australia, that a great deal of volunteer work is done by older Australians who are still active (DeVaus, Gray & Stanton, 2003; Warburton & McLaughlin, 2005). How to support older people who become frail with chronic illnesses, either physical and/or mental, will then be considered in a section entitled 'supported living'. The last section, 'dying, death and bereavement', covers the highest amount of compensation required for meeting needs as the older person dies.

Independent living

This section begins with an introduction to Sarah Atwood, because at this stage in her life she is still firmly in control and deserves to have the first hearing.

Ms Sarah Atwood lives in the small rural town of Bushnut. She has lived here for 10 years now. One of her daughters persuaded her to move nearer to her and the grandchildren and then promptly left because her husband got a job in Sydney. Sarah doesn't mind as she has four children and many grandchildren who are scattered across Australia. Several of her children are always treating her to plane tickets and pleasant holidays with her grandchildren and great-grandchildren. Caroline, her eldest daughter, lives an hour away, and they meet up regularly. The neighbours are great, and she usually feeds their cat while they are away and gets to chat with Sally across the back fence when hanging out the washing. Tom, her neighbour's husband, is always offering to do little jobs around the house, but Sarah prefers to pay someone to do it.

Every morning Sarah walks to a local café to buy a cup of coffee and have a chat with the young girls and other regulars. She then buys her daily provisions, which always include fresh protein and vegetables. Playing bowls has been her lifesaver, and the club is just a kilometre down the road – she is in the women's team (over 70s), and they meet for a game every Monday and Friday afternoon. On Fridays a few of them stay at the club for tea, and she takes the courtesy bus home – Stan the driver is a gentleman and always walks her to the door and waits until she has her key in the lock before leaving. On Tuesdays she visits a friend at the local residential aged care facility, where she used to be a volunteer. The other day a group in the day room had a discussion about living wills, and later, after much thought, Sarah discussed this with her eldest son. He then arranged to visit next month to get it organised with her solicitor. Sarah keeps her house and patio as neat as a pin and, being a lifetime member of the Country Women's Association, she cooks the lightest sponge cakes for their fundraisers. One or other of the children phone her each night, and by the time she has finished talking it is time to settle contentedly in front of the television.

When winter arrives, Sarah will make an appointment at the local health centre for her 'check-up', as she calls it. There will be her free 'flu' injection, and she will ask the nurse about her hearing because the kids say she is deaf. She will not mention the stress incontinence that she has, because that is just between her and the chemist and is not a big problem. The nurse will weigh her and she will be delighted that she has not put on any weight (hasn't lost any either but at least the eating is now well under control). Catherine, the nurse, will try to get her to go to 'geri gym', but she will avoid that one. Sarah will ask if they have a cure for arthritis yet (her little joke!), and if not she will keep 'popping the pills'. If she sees the doctor, she will tell him about her swollen ankles. She will probably encourage her friend Amy to make an appointment (she always avoids the doctor) at the same time so that she can get a lift.

How old is she? 80 years young!

Sarah's story is fictional, but it is an example of someone ageing in place – in touch with enough people to keep her connected and reasonably content with life, where she still makes a contribution and in return receives kindly help in the community. Reading between the lines, it is reasonable to guess her needs are associated with transport, access to health services and advice regarding self-management of her stress incontinence and pain associated with arthritis. Access, health promotion and transport are all included as major problems in the Australian report on aged care in rural, regional and remote Australia (National Rural Health Alliance [NRHA], 2005), so Sarah's situation is reasonably typical.

Despite government incentives to improve health services in rural and regional Australia (Humphreys, Wakerman & Wells, 2006), it is undoubtedly the case that older people in rural areas become increasingly dependent on the goodwill of the community for socialising and transport. Such support is more readily available to people who have the privilege of longevity in their local area, with friends and family close by. The people who fall through the gaps are those who have more recently arrived. Although it is not officially a *quid pro quo* system, people moving to a rural location have a lot to gain by becoming involved with the community and finding out what it has to offer and what they can offer in return. Nurses and other health professionals who live in the community can, by virtue of their professional standing, help keep this fellowship alive by modelling citizenship, joining in both informal and formal community organisations, and in particular welcoming newcomers.

Regular conversations with the family are a great way of monitoring an older person's wellbeing. Sarah's daughters can always tell if she is getting a bit sad and needs someone to visit for a short time and perhaps take her to stay with another sibling – this usually happens during the winter. It is a well-established fact that depression is underdiagnosed in the older population (Byrne & Neville, 2010). Modern technology is fast becoming an essential part of older people's lives, especially for staying in touch with family members and friends living far away. It is also useful for accessing health information and keeping the brain agile (Greenhalgh et al., 2013).

Useful website:

Health assessment for people aged 75 years and older in Australia
http://www.health.gov.au/internet/main/publishing.nsf/Content/mbsprimarycare_mbsitem_75andolder

Please access the fact sheet on the above website and note the component parts of the assessment.

Full health assessments for people aged 75 years and older are the most proactive ways for health professionals to engage with older people who are well. The assessments provide an opportunity for the older person and the health professionals to take stock of the situation and make plans for maintaining optimum health and function. Sarah's approach to her health is based on common sense and, while this has served her well, it is now time for her to undergo a thorough assessment so that issues can be picked up well before they develop into a number of problems that could compromise her wellbeing.

It is quite common for medical practitioners to delegate some of the health assessment for people aged 75 years and older to nurses. Components of the health assessment are:

- information collection (history, physical examination and tests)
- making an overall assessment
- recommending appropriate interventions and adapting them to the person
- giving health information and advice
- keeping records of the health assessment and offering to share these with the older person and (following discussion with the health team and the patient) with an appropriate other (e.g. close friend or relative).

In addition, health professionals are asked to consider whether the person is eating well, has good oral and dental health, and whether they are socially isolated or in need of community services (Department of Health and Ageing [DoHA], n.d.).

When Sarah made her planned visit to the health centre, as mentioned above, the nurse recommended that she take advantage of the full assessment and offered her an appointment at home. From then onwards, Sarah had an assessment each year.

Sarah's swollen ankles were due to mild heart failure so she started taking an antihypertensive and diuretic; she also had a referral to a dietician to help her plan to lose 5 kg during the next year. The nurse provided education about the new tablets and the management of her stress incontinence. She also gave Sarah a useful leaflet that included a web address that Sarah and her daughter used to look up the tablets and their side effects. Sarah was also advised by the nurse to keep a record of the pain she experienced from the arthritis, and when she saw the daily pattern, Sarah chose to take the tablets regularly twice a day.

At this stage people are usually in control of their own lives, making their own decisions and accepting responsibility to stay well and safe, if only to avoid becoming a 'burden' to family or friends. The nurse and other health professionals should be mindful not to disrupt the pattern of self-care that the person and their support network have set up. They achieve this by being non-judgemental and having respect for other people's values and choices. In the supportive educative system, the nurse assesses the situation and provides the person with information to make decisions. A nurse with a sound knowledge of the primary health services available can ensure that the older person is accessing every possible support to maintain optimum health.

Primary health services in rural communities are part of the Department of Health and Ageing's Rural Primary Health Services Program. These services are specifically designed to improve access to programs that promote wellness. The categories 'regional centre', 'rural' and 'remote' show a range of services available to the community, which include clinics where patients attend, outreach services where health professionals visit the community to provide services, and telemedicine. These services are not uniform – they change with government funding, workforce availability and location. Therefore, it is important that nurses keep up-to-date information for older people and their supporters.

It is easier for older people to preserve their identity and standing in smaller communities than in urban areas, where there is less community mindedness. Astute nurses do hear how older people are faring and encourage support for older people within the community. Chatting to people at work and engaging in the community are informal ways of entering into the spirit of the community.

Supported living

The reality is that people in their 80s and 90s have a higher incidence of chronic illnesses (e.g. cancer, arthritis, diabetes, heart failure) than younger persons. These illnesses, while they can be managed, may begin to take a heavy toll on the older person's functioning and wellbeing.

This is particularly the case when more illnesses and symptoms accumulate, adding to the complexity of the management of the older person's condition. Below are two quotes from an elderly person who contributed to a study on the experience of chronic illness in rural Australia (FitzGerald, 1995, p. 144):

> I find exercise is the biggest factor that can drop my blood sugar, if I've … [pause] … the level. Now the trouble is with the arthritis often I am so sore that I can't exercise.

> … I was previously on a gout diet, an arthritis diet, on a weight loss diet and now on a diabetic diet – and that left me with about a lettuce leaf to eat.

These quotes are examples of the frustrations associated with multiple pathology and the limits of self-care.

The government has made chronic illnesses a national priority, and these include asthma, cancer, cardiovascular health, diabetes, injury prevention, mental health, arthritis and musculoskeletal conditions, and dementia (Australian Institute of Health and Welfare [AIHW], 2013a). Of note, Aboriginal and Torres Strait Islander people are over-represented in each of these conditions (DoHA, 2010a), which will reduce their life expectancy and quality of life in later years. There is an Indigenous Chronic Disease Package, as part of the 'Closing the Gap' program (DoHA, 2013), that includes supplementary services (DoHA, 2010b).

With chronic illnesses, as one illness impacts on another, self-care becomes increasingly arduous for the older person. Increasing medical problems may mean that the older person needs more help. They may find that their medicines interact or have unwanted side effects; they may also find that they are at risk of becoming sad or depressed and may encounter social isolation and even suffer financial difficulties.

Referral to a geriatrician gives the older person access to one specialist who will provide a holistic service and take into account multiple pathologies, as well as the person's wishes and social context. Well-established general practitioners (GPs) in rural communities are very experienced at dealing with the problems associated with multiple chronic illnesses (chronic and complex care) and ageing in rural areas; with the backing of a team of nurses with specialist knowledge, these GPs can provide an excellent service to frail older people still living at home. However, this is not always the case in rural areas where there are workforce problems. As function declines in the older person living in rural Australia, the problems associated with access and transport are exacerbated (NRHA, 2005). In particular, rural areas are underserviced because of shortages of doctors and allied health personnel.

In the partially compensatory care system, carers are very important as care agents – and this is where single older people are particularly vulnerable. A range of services is available that will help enable frail older people to stay at home. The Australian Government has provided a national information service, which is available both online and by telephone. This is an important service for rural communities because there may be more on offer than might be expected. This includes support for the carers in terms of both finance and any help required to fulfil the self-care needs of the older person (Orem as cited in Pearson et al., 2005).

Respite care is also available to allow carers a break. Each community through
its historical evolution has different providers who broker services for aged care
packages. Again this makes it important for nurses to know their community and
the variety of services available to support older people. Many communities have
Community Aged Care Packages (CACPs) and Extended Aged Care at Home
(EACH) packages available. Some of these can be specific for clients with dementia (DoHA, 2012). Distance is often a disadvantage to clients using these services,
as hours of travel often diminish the hours of care provided in the packages to
people living out of town or a considerable distance from the service provider.

The first step in arranging more support is to ask for an assessment by
an Aged Care Assessment Team (ACAT, or Aged Care Assessment Service
[ACAS] in Victoria). This assessment of the older person's daily living activities identifies the needs and matches them with available services as part of the
Health and Community Care (HACC) program. In the first instance, the service required may be domestic help with meals, community transport, cleaning
and/or shopping. There are also services for personal hygiene, medication, in-
jections and dressing changes.

Time has passed and Sarah is feeling her age now – 87 years old. She had
a fall three winters ago and lay on the floor for four hours before Sally from
next door heard her shouting. Sarah had a hip replacement but really has not
been able to walk far since, and besides she seems to have lost her nerve
and zest for life. Her ankles are swollen and she is only comfortable wearing
slippers. She has daily help from a professional carer who assists her with the
housework, shopping and getting dressed. The kids still phone and visit but she
won't travel to go and see them now. The family pays Sally to take her a cooked
meal three times a week. Sarah is picked up once a week and spends five hours
at the Day Centre. Here she gets some rehabilitation and social interaction but
comes home exhausted after an hour in the minibus. Her medicines come in
packs from the pharmacy each Monday, and she follows the instructions carefully.
She has stopped using the computer and really only has visitors when her
daughter, Mary, who lives locally, comes to stay each month. She doesn't mind
too much; she is very tired and dozes much of the day with her feet up. The
family are bickering about how much she can do on her own and whether she
should go into a nursing home and where that should be. Sarah just agrees with
each of them and hopes she doesn't have to make the decision.

VIGNETTE CONTINUED

The Australian Government supports 'Ageing in Place' (AIHW, 2013b), and the Foundation for Rural and Regional Renewal (FRRR) offers grants for innovative projects to accommodate this initiative (2013). Successful projects include window replacement, storage sheds for mobility scooters and installation of automatic doors. The projects are practical and evidence of good ideas that can be generated locally. The website lists all the projects and is well worth reviewing in order to appreciate the great work that is being done on the ground (FRRR, 2013).

Most larger rural towns have some accommodation for retirees, such as independent living units and low-level care facilities. They usually have features that help people who are becoming less mobile (e.g. wheelchair access and small raised garden beds) to remain in their own homes and keep active and engaged with hobbies. These may or may not be connected to other services for older people, such as communal space, community activities and meals. There may also be accommodation for higher levels of care culminating in full care (total compensatory care). Whether people decide to accept this type of accommodation at an early stage when they are still reasonably independent or decide to live in their own homes, with adaptations made as necessary, is a personal choice. The former means that they do not have to make difficult decisions later when they are frail and may find it difficult to process all the information required to make a difficult choice. They also remain in one community near friends. Residential aged care facilities (RACF) tend to be in town, and the one nearest to the older person may well be full when they decide to move. Therefore, it is sometimes the case that older people have to leave their community to find a place in a RACF, and this compounds their sense of loss. It is important to remember that the majority of older people do not live in RACFs, preferring to remain at home with high levels of support (Hatcher, 2010).

VIGNETTE CONTINUED

John, the eldest son, came up to stay for a few days and, together with Sarah and Mary, sat down and looked through the advanced care directive that had been written years earlier. Together they decided to look at either the local nursing home or the one that is located near Mary. This will enable Sarah to stay in the region and be visited regularly by Mary. The documents really helped them make the decision, as some of the children wanted Sarah to move to a city where she would have access to more medical services. Sarah had firmly stated earlier that she did not want to become dependent on her children, nor did she want to have aggressive medical treatment – and this is still her firmly held desire. The original decision she made at the age of 60 years – to move to the region – had turned out to be a good one. She had lived there for 28 years and had no regrets.

Increasing dependence can be an unhappy time for the older person, who may worry about becoming a burden on friends and family. However, it can also be a time of increasing peacefulness – letting go of the bustle of community life. Each person deserves to be respected for how they choose to adapt to changes in their abilities; alterations in mood and motivation should not be read as a sign of mental health problems or forgetfulness seen as a sign of dementia. Alternatively, it is a time when a person is susceptible to depression and may display signs of dementia. Health professionals who engage with older people are trained to unobtrusively notice signs of depression and dementia.

Dying, death and bereavement

There is no uniform sequence of growing dependency before death; indeed, most older people are still living at home when they die. The longer people live, however, the more likely it is that they will receive end-of-life care in either a regional hospital or RACF. The leading causes of death in Australia are ischaemic heart disease, cerebrovascular diseases, dementia and Alzheimer's disease (Australian Bureau of Statistics, 2013). Palliative care is covered in Chapter 5.

Dying can be a prolonged process where there is time for a full assessment and planning for palliative care, or it can be sudden as the result of an accident and/or acute episode of illness such as a stroke. Advanced care directives and documents of power of attorney can prevent people receiving inappropriate care and treatment in these instances, but only if they are known to exist. Increasingly, RACFs will not transfer older people to hospital for treatment if they know it is the older person's wishes not to do so and they have the support of their next of kin (Jeong, Higgins & McMillan, 2010). This is a very difficult or impossible decision to make in an emergency situation and results in transfers that can be detrimental to the older person's physical, mental and social wellbeing.

Palliative care and care of the dying person and their carers can be planned for periods of as little as a day or for several months (Johnson & Chang, 2014). It involves a holistic assessment, selection of appropriate interventions, implementation of the interventions and evaluation. Community nurses in rural areas can provide these services depending on where the person resides. However, this is not usually a 24-hour service providing total care. Often, larger towns will provide a visiting palliative care service that can give specialist advice to the community nurses and family who provide day-to-day care for the older person. Live-in carers such as partners or children are invaluable in the implementation of the plan. Caring for anyone dying at home is a considerable undertaking, and it should be remembered that the partner of an older person may be frail and elderly too, and children may be unwell or elderly themselves (Kenny, Hall, Zapart & Davis, 2010).

Useful websites:

Australian Government Department of Health website for palliative care
http://www.health.gov.au/palliativecare

Educational materials for palliative care
http://www.palliativecare.org.au/Agedcare/Agedcareresources.aspx

Sarah lived in the RACF for just under a year. She had a stroke on Monday morning and died peacefully on Wednesday afternoon with Mary at her bedside. During these last few days she was visited by the palliative care team and, together with Mary and the staff of the RACF, an 'end-of-life plan was initiated'. Mary was very relieved that she and John were both involved in the process of writing Sarah's advanced care directive and felt that her last days were full of care rather than struggle.

She is buried in the town she called home. Sally and the children put wild flowers on her grave once a year.

While some people would regard death at a 'ripe old age' to be a normal stage in our evolution, attention needs to be given to those left behind – particularly elderly partners who may be alone for the first time in their lives. Besides the grief that those left behind are suffering, it may be that couples compensate for each other in a number of ways. It is not unusual for an elderly partner to sink into depression and/or lose function following the death of their loved one. Besides being helped and supported by the rural community, it is best practice that grieving partners are encouraged by health professionals to have their yearly health assessments or medical appointments, and time should be provided during these sessions to talk about their bereavement and the changes that have eventuated (Naef, Ward, Mahrer-Imhof & Grande, 2013).

Summary

In this chapter, we have covered:

- the perspective of older people in a rural community whenever possible
- positive attitudes to living well and living longer that enable older people to lead healthy, active lives

- chronic diseases that can adversely affect the wellbeing of older people
- the joint effort of lay carers and health professionals to assist elderly people with care needs in the community
- planning ahead and discussing attitudes to old age and dying as constructive ways of ensuring that clients receive their preference for treatment.

Reflective questions

1 In what ways do nurses contribute to community spirit and wellbeing?
2 How do older people contribute to the wellbeing of your community?
3 How much are nurses considered to be leaders in your community?
4 In what ways can nurses demonstrate leadership in their community?
5 In what ways are nurses able to demonstrate respect for older people in the community?
6 What aged care packages are available in your own community?
7 How can a nurse encourage older people to consider making advanced care directives without causing offence?

References

Australian Bureau of Statistics (ABS). (2013). *Causes of death, Australia, 2011*, Catalogue No. 3303.0. Canberra: ABS. Retrieved September 4, 2013, from http://www.abs.gov.au/ausstats/abs@.nsf/Lookup/3303.0Chapter42011

Australian Institute of Health and Welfare (AIHW). (2013a). Chronic diseases. Canberra: AIHW. Retrieved September 4, 2013, from http://www.aihw.gov.au/chronic-diseases/

——. (2013b). The desire to age in place among older Australians. Bulletin no. 114. cat. no. AUS 169. Canberra: AIHW. Retrieved November 28, 2013, from http://www.aihw.gov.au/WorkArea/DownloadAsset.aspx?id=60129543248

Byrne, G. & Neville, C. (2010). *Community mental health for older people*. Sydney: Elsevier Australia.

De Vaus, D., Gray, M. & Stanton, D. (2003). Measuring the value of unpaid household, caring and voluntary work of older Australians. Research Paper No. 34. Melbourne: Australian Institute of Family Studies. Retrieved September 4, 2013, from http://www.aifs.gov.au/institute/pubs/respaper/RP34.pdf

Department of Health and Ageing (DoHA). (n.d.). Health assessment for people aged 75 years and older [Factsheet]. Canberra: DoHA. Retrieved September 4, 2013, from http://www.health.gov.au/internet/main/publishing.nsf/Content/mbsprimarycare_mbsitem_75andolder

———. (2010a). Closing the gap: Tackling Indigenous chronic disease. Canberra: DoHA. Retrieved November 28, 2013, from http://www.health.gov.au/tackling-chronic-disease

———. (2010b). Care coordination and supplementary services program. Canberra: DoHA. Retrieved November 28, 2013, from http://www.health.gov.au/internet/ctg/publishing.nsf/Content/practice-detail-card-10-care-coordination-and-supplementary-services-program/$file/DHA0002.9%20A4%20Practice%20Detail%20Card%2010%20CCSS%20WEB.pdf

———. (2012). Commonwealth HACC Program. Retrieved June 3, 2013, from http://www.health.gov.au/internet/main/publishing.nsf/Content/hacc-vindex.htm

———. (2013). Indigenous chronic disease package. [Factsheet]. Retrieved November 28, 2013, from http://www.health.gov.au/internet/ctg/publishing.nsf/Content/Indigenous-Chronic-Disease-Package-factsheet

FitzGerald, M. (1995). The experience of chronic illness in rural Australia (Unpublished PhD thesis). University of New England, Armidale, NSW.

Foundation for Rural and Regional Renewal (FRRR). (2013). Innovative projects help rural people age in place. Retrieved November 28, 2013, from (http://www.frrr.org.au/cb_pages/news/Innovative_CARA_projects_help_rural_people_age_in_place.php

Greenhalgh, T., Wherton, J., Sugarhood, P., Hinder, S., Procter, R. & Stones, R. (2013). What matters to older people with assisted living needs? A phenomenological analysis of the use and non-use of telehealth and telecare. *Social Science & Medicine*, 93, 86–94. Retrieved September 4, 2013, from http://dx.doi.org/10.1016/j.socscimed.2013.05.036

Hatcher, D. (2010). Holding momentum: A grounded theory study of older persons sustaining living at home (Unpublished PhD thesis). University of Western Sydney, Australia. Retrieved June 3, 2013, from http://arrow.uws.edu.au:8080/vital/access/manager/Repository/uws:8964

Humphreys, J. S., Wakerman, J. & Wells, R. (2006). What do we mean by sustainable rural health services? Implications for rural health research. *Australian Journal of Rural Health*, 14(1), 33–5. doi: 10.1111/j.1440–1584.2006.00750.x

Jeong, S. Y., Higgins, I. & McMillan, M. (2010). The essentials of advance care planning for end-of-life care for older people. *Journal of Clinical Nursing*, 19, 389–97. doi: 10.1111/j.1365–2702.2009.03001.x

Johnson, A. & Chang, E. (2014). *Caring for older people in Australia: Principles for nursing practice*. Milton, Qld: Wiley.

Kenny, P. M., Hall, J. P., Zapart, S. & Davis, P. R. (2010). Informal care and home-based palliative care: The health-related quality of life of carers. *Journal of Pain and Symptom Management*, 40(1), 35–48. doi: http://dx.doi.org/10.1016/j.jpainsymman.2009.11.322

Naef, R., Ward, R., Mahrer-Imhof, R. & Grande, G. (2013). Characteristics of the bereavement experience of older persons after spousal loss: An integrative review.

International Journal of Nursing Studies, 50(8), 1108–21. doi: http://dx.doi.
org/10.1016/j.ijnurstu.2012.11.026

National Rural Health Alliance (NRHA). (2005). *Older people and aged care in rural,
regional and remote Australia*. Melbourne: NRHA & ACSA. Retrieved September
4, 2013, from http://www.agedcare.org.au/what-we-do/policies-and-position/
policies-pdfs/Rural_remote_policy05.pdf

Pearson, A., Vaughan, B. & FitzGerald, M. (2005). *Nursing models for practice*
(3rd ed.). Sydney: Butterworth-Heinemann.

Warburton, J. & McLaughlin, D. (2005). 'Lots of little kindnesses': Valuing the role
of older Australians as informal volunteers in the community. *Ageing and Society*,
25(5), 715–30. doi: 10.1017/S0144686X05003648

9 Mental health in rural communities

Margaret McLeod and Sally Drummond

Learning objectives   On completion of this chapter, the reader will be able to:

- understand the rural environment and its relationship to mental health and wellbeing

- discuss attitudes towards mental illness in the rural context

- identify mental health matters from a lifespan approach

- acknowledge the roles of rural generalist nurses/midwives and mental health specialists within interdisciplinary teams

- understand that rural people are faced with particular challenges when accessing mental health information and services and recognise the specific needs of Indigenous Australians.

Key words   Interdisciplinary teams, mental ill-health, stigma, contemporary models of care, access and equity

Chapter overview

This chapter provides an overview of mental health and wellbeing in rural Australia. The narrative will be guided by a lifespan approach exploring health promotion, information, and access and equity with respect to mental health services for children, adolescents, youth, adults and older adults. The specific healthcare needs of Australia's Aboriginal and Torres Strait Islander people will also be addressed. The chapter covers current trends, models of care available to individuals experiencing mental ill-health, and the roles of generalist nurses/midwives, mental health clinicians and other interdisciplinary team members. Collectively, they aim to support rural healthcare users to help them achieve their individual goals, with additional support from family members and significant others.

Trends in mental ill-health in rural Australia

The health and wellbeing of rural people, which includes mental health, are priorities for interdisciplinary healthcare professionals who work in many parts of Australia. In 2000, the Commonwealth's Department of Health and Aged Care defined mental health as 'the capacity of individuals and groups to inter-act with one another and their environment in ways that promote subjective wellbeing, optimal development and use of mental abilities ...' (p. 3).

Unfortunately, rurality is often linked to a reduction in access (and there-fore equity) to a range of health promotion activities, information, services and clinical providers, with these deficits affecting mental healthcare pro-vision. In Australia, one in five people will experience a significant mental health problem at some stage of their life (Petrie, 2011). In 2007, the Aus-tralian Government collected national survey data relating to anxiety, mood and substance use disorders. The data, representing individuals aged 16–85 years, were subsequently published in the *National Survey of Mental Health and Wellbeing* (Australian Bureau of Statistics [ABS], 2007). See the following web link for prevalence rates of selected mental illnesses across the lifespan (Department of Health and Ageing, 2009, p. 16):

<http://www.health.gov.au/internet/main/publishing.nsf/Content/9A5A0E8BDFC5 5D3BCA257BF0001C1B1C/$File/plan09v2.pdf>

It should be noted that individuals with a mental illness are more likely to experience physical comorbidities. Therefore, it is important for all rural cli-nicians to be aware of mental health issues and the specialist services that are available locally, those delivered from regional hubs or those situated in distant metropolitan areas.

The ABS (2007) states that 'mental illness is the largest single cause of disability in Australia, accounting for nearly 30 per cent of the burden of non-fatal disease' (as cited in Hungerford et al., 2012, p. 2). Not surprisingly, given the extent of this burden, mental health is now one of the national health priorities for the Australian Government (Beaton, Mann & Grigg, 2011). Therefore, the need for rural clinicians (including nurses and midwives) to be aware of mental illness, its diagnosis and treatment is paramount. There will be no escaping the responsibility in the rural context of caring for individuals with a mental illness and acknowledging that they are particularly vulnerable, with some remaining undiagnosed or undertreated for years or a lifetime. As Happell, Cowin, Roper, Lakeman and Cox (2013) attest, 'nurses [and midwives] will find themselves working with people experiencing mental illness and mental health challenges, regardless of the setting in which they choose to practise' (p. 391).

In Australia, mental ill-health is usually referred to under the broad banner of mental illness. However, other common terms – including mental disorder and mental dysfunction – are used in some Mental Health Acts, reflecting the legislative frameworks of particular states and territories. Hungerford et al. (2012) urge caution in the use of appropriate language when communicating with people who are experiencing mental ill-health, as some terms or labels have the potential to be disempowering rather than empowering (p. 7).

Often people experiencing mental ill-health are stigmatised by others. Stigma can be defined as 'an attribute, behaviour or reputation that is perceived, constructed and/or represented by a group of people, society or culture in a negative way' (Hungerford et al., 2012, p. 8). It can lead to loss of employment, homelessness, family and social isolation, poor self-esteem and distress (Hungerford et al., 2012). In Australia, the work of organisations such as *beyondblue*, SANE Australia and headspace have resulted in 'improved community perceptions' following education and involvement of communities (Hungerford et al., 2012, p. 8). This is particularly important in rural locations, where community members are more likely to encounter a range of significant challenges including floods, storms, fires, cyclones and prolonged drought (Australian Centre for Posttraumatic Mental Health, *beyondblue*, Australian Centre for Grief and Bereavement, & Australian Red Cross, 2011). Some townships have assumed responsibility for educating specific target groups, including middle-aged and older men, with Men's Sheds and Pitstop initiatives. Further, local service clubs such as Rotary are used to communicate mental health information and service entry points, particularly when natural events or disasters lead to financial hardship.

All members of interdisciplinary health teams, including mental health specialists, must be mindful of their own power and prejudices, which could further propagate stigma in rural communities. Munro and Baker (2007) identify six behaviours attributed to health professionals when 'caring' for mental health consumers:

- talking about consumers rather than to consumers
- putting down and ridiculing consumers

- failing to provide information to consumers to enable them to make informed decisions
- failing to provide appropriate or respectful services
- failing to respect the information provided to the service by family members
- perpetuating negative stereotypes.

Children and adolescents

In Australia, 14–20% of children and adolescents experience mental health problems, with boys being more highly represented than girls (Hungerford et al., 2012, p. 15). Of particular significance are anxiety disorders, which are more common in females than in males (Reavley, Allen, Jorm, Morgan & Purcell, 2010). Anxiety disorders include separation anxiety and depression. Some children may have behavioural disorders where socially unacceptable conduct is displayed. These children are often identified as troubled or troublemakers (WHO Collaborating Centre for Evidence in Mental Health Policy, 2004). A child with oppositional defiant disorder, for example, may present as disobedient, provocative and defiant. In the later adolescent age group, bipolar disorder, schizophrenia, depression, suicidal thoughts and high-risk behaviours (including smoking or drug use) are more commonly present (Hungerford et al., 2012).

Correspondingly, there has been a commitment for many years for early intervention services for children that focus on physical, social and psychological health. A number of government policies have incorporated the principle of early intervention, including 'the National Mental Health Policy, the National Action Plan for Promotion, Prevention and Early Intervention for Mental Health and Partners in Prevention – Mental Health and General Practice 2004' (Happell et al., 2013, p. 91). One of the original Australian intervention programs was the Early Psychosis and Prevention Intervention Centre (EPPIC). Its core aim was to reduce treatment delays for young people with early psychosis. Barry and Jenkins (2007) suggest that a range of interventions may 'help prevent a major decline in a person's biological, social and psychological state that may occur after a psychotic episode in a young person's formative years' (as cited in Happell et al., 2013, p. 91).

There are specific child and adolescent mental health services throughout Australia, with much of the care taking place in primary healthcare settings – for example, headspace.

headspace – National Youth Mental Health Foundation
http://www.headspace.org.au/

Adults

In Australia, young adults in the 18–24 years age range are the largest group with mental health issues (Mindframe National Media Initiative, as cited in Hungerford et al., 2012, p. 15). While some individuals enter adulthood with an existing mental illness, others may develop an illness in the course of their lifetimes. The Mental Health Acts for each state and territory provide a legislative framework for care and treatment, guided by the principles of the least-restrictive environment (Elder, Evans & Nizette, 2013). This means that individuals receiving mental health care should remain in their homes or communities when it is deemed safe for them, their families or others, rather than in voluntary or involuntary mental health facilities.

> Please become familiar with the Mental Health Act in your state or territory
> as legislation and terminology differ. This information can be sourced on
> state and territory government health websites.

Older people

Although Australia's population is ageing, many people will live healthy, independent lifestyles (Hungerford et al., 2012). However, the fastest growing age group is 85 years and above, which equates to 1.8% of the total population (Elder et al., 2013), and people in this age group are more likely to have a number of physical health issues or disabilities. According to Garlick and Koch (2011), 'the most distinctive symptom of older adults over younger is the existence of multiple comorbid disorders' (p. 252). It is therefore important for health professionals to be aware of the specific needs of this age group, including mental health and mental ill-health considerations. This is particularly important in rural communities, which have disproportionate levels of older unsupported people, given that younger inhabitants need to exodus small townships to access education or find employment.

Older people are at greater risk of anxiety and depression. In Australia, over two million people experience anxiety each year, affecting on average one in three women and one in five men (*beyondblue*, 2013b). In contrast, 'around one million Australian adults have depression [with] on average one in eight men and one in five women' experiencing depression in their lifetime (ABS, as cited in Jorm, Allen, Morgan, Ryan & Purcell, 2013, p. 5). Further, 'dementia affects around 5 per cent of people aged over 65 years, and approximately 20 per cent of those over 80 years of age', with one-third experiencing moderate to severe behavioural and psychiatric symptoms (ABS, as cited in Hungerford et al., 2012, p. 416). The first challenge for health professionals working with older people is to set aside preconceived ideas and to acknowledge the unique-ness of each individual (Hungerford et al., 2012). Thereafter, they should be ready to actively listen, without judgement, while undertaking the assessment process. Clinicians should be mindful that each person is the product of 'a com-plex interaction of diverse influences', including psychological, sociological and biological components (Hungerford et al., 2012, p. 421). Taking these factors into account, the health professional should be ready to commit to a person-centred approach to the initial assessment and any care that follows, further allowing health professionals to embrace a culturally responsive framework.

The assessment and diagnosis of a mental illness in an older person is a complex task requiring the expertise of a specialist such as a psychogeriatri-cian, in addition to other interdisciplinary team members. Depression is com-mon in older people, including those in aged care facilities, but it may not be acknowledged by the person or identified by health professionals, leading to it being missed and therefore ignored (Jorm et al., 2013; Hungerford et al., 2012). Older people may not fit into the strict criteria of a major depressive episode, but disabling symptoms could include hopelessness, lack of concentration, despair, sadness, withdrawal, reduced pleasure in things or suicidal thoughts (*beyondblue*, 2013a). It should be noted that suicide rates in elderly males are comparable to suicide rates in younger males, making this a particular concern (De Leo & Ormskerk, 1991; Szanto et al., 2002; WHO, as cited in Hungerford et al., 2012, p. 436). The most effective way to assess for depression is by inter-viewing the older person. The clinician may also use an assessment tool such as the geriatric depression scale (GDS) prior to introducing one or more treatment regimes (Garlick & Koch, 2011).

One reliable cognitive assessment tool is the Mini Mental State Examina-tion (MMSE). At its most basic level, the MMSE involves 'testing orientation to time, place and person, and short- and long-term recall, in an unstructured way' (Plakiotis & O'Connor, 2012, p. 621). However, the MMSE does have limitations, 'particularly in appraising frontal lobe functions such as complex planning skills', with this deficit leading to the development of a range of new cognitive screening tools (Plakiotis & O'Connor, 2012, p. 621). In older adults, it is important to distinguish between delirium and dementia as the presentations can be similar. According to Tschanz et al. (2000), several criteria distinguish delirium from dementia:

- state of consciousness
- stability
- duration
- rate of onset
- cause (as cited in Kneisl, Wilson & Trigoboff, 2004, p. 238).

If treated promptly and appropriately, delirium can be reversed – for example, a urinary tract infection could be treated with antibiotics.

The most widely used assessment tool, which is used for all age groups, is the Mental State Examination (MSE). The common way for MSE information to be gathered is by means of an interview between the healthcare provider and the service user (Happell et al., 2013; Gaynor, Harder, Munro & Robins, 2011). The mental status assessment is usually based on observations and questions asked during the interview. According to Elder et al. (2009), the interview is semi-structured and aims to 'assess a client's neurological and psychological status across several domains, such as perception, affect, thought content, thought form and speech' (as cited in Gaynor et al., 2011, p. 29). Pederson (2005) provides further details by identifying eight categories that guide the healthcare provider during the course of the interview and later when writing up the descriptors of each category:

- general appearance
- behaviour/activity
- speech and language
- mood and affect
- thought process and content
- perceptual disturbances
- memory/cognition
- judgement and insight (p. 36).

For example, in the descriptor for 'appearance', the healthcare provider may have observed and noted that the person was dirty and dishevelled, scantily clad despite the cold weather and presenting a downturned head, resulting in limited eye contact.

Aboriginal and Torres Strait Islander Australians

There are approximately 517 200 Aboriginal and Torres Strait Islander Australians, representing 2.5% of the total population (West, Usher, Thompson & Spurgeon, 2011). The mental health and social and emotional wellbeing of Aboriginal and Torres Strait Islander people require special consideration, for they encapsulate a number of aspects, including the physical, social, emotional, spiritual and cultural wellbeing of the whole community (Jorm et al., 2013). Evidence suggests that much of the stress faced by Aboriginal and Torres Strait Islander Australians is centred around the ongoing impact of colonisation and the resilience required to combat challenges of continued and sustained trauma (Eckermann et al., 2010, p. 84). Contributing to these stressors are the increased levels of discrimination and prejudice, the identified increase in poverty and economic insecurity for Aboriginal and Torres Strait Islander communities and individuals, as well as the over-representation of Aboriginal and Torres Strait Islander people within correctional facilities (Eckermann et al., 2010, p. 84). Mental ill-health and suicide rates for many Aboriginal and Torres Strait Islander communities are also a recognised concern for the Australian Government and, more importantly, for the Aboriginal and Torres Strait Islander communities that, as health professionals, you will be working alongside as culturally responsive practitioners.

Aboriginal and Torres Strait Islander mental health workers play a vital role in supporting Aboriginal and Torres Strait Islander Australians when they access mental health services. Aboriginal and Torres Strait Islander health workers are better placed to determine the specific mental health issues of their peoples and what is required to access culturally safe care (Jorm et al., 2013). Some workers have completed training in mental health and psychological therapies, and their diverse roles include 'case management, screening, assessment, referrals, transport to and attendance at specialist appointments, education, improving access to mainstream services, advocacy, counselling, support for family and acute distress response' (Jorm et al., 2013, p. 7).

Non-Indigenous health professionals must recognise that Aboriginal and Torres Strait Islander Australians believe that 'good health is holistic and defined by the harmony that exists between individuals, communities and the universe' (Booth & Carroll, as cited in Hunter, Gill & Toombs,

2013, p. 207). This belief system needs to be considered when providing culturally sensitive and responsive, individualised, holistic care to Aboriginal and Torres Strait Islander Australians. Still, Hunter et al. (2013) warn that, given the diversity across Aboriginal and Torres Strait Islander populations in Australia, there is no single right or appropriate way of communicating with Aboriginal and Torres Strait Islander people: 'it is perhaps more important to be confident about the integrity and respect you bring to the clinical encounter' (p. 210).

In the mental health context, health professionals use advanced observation and communication skills when gathering and later recording MSE data (Happell et al., 2013). However, it must be acknowledged that 'the MSE is strongly culturally determined, being based on a white Anglo-Saxon Protestant (WASP) understanding of what is normal and what might be considered a mental, social or emotional disturbance' (Happell et al., 2013, p. 358). Therefore, extreme caution must be afforded when assessing an Aboriginal and Torres Strait Islander Australian – or anyone, for that matter, from another cultural group – as it is easy 'to judge someone as disordered when we have not reflected on how our own cultural identity, position, life-world and world-view might be influencing our clinical judgement' (Happell et al., 2013, p. 358).

Useful websites:

beyondblue
http://www.beyondblue.org.au
http://www.beyondblue.org.au/resources
http://www.youthbeyondblue.com/

thedesk
http://www.thedesk.org.au/

mindhealthconnect
http://www.mindhealthconnect.org.au

MoodGYM
http://www.moodgym.anu.edu.au

EPPIC
http://www.eppic.org.au

SANE Australia
http://www.sane.org

Australian Institute of Health and Welfare
http://www.aihw.gov.au/
http://www.aihw.gov.au/mentalhealth/indix.cfm

Trent is 16 years of age and is currently enrolled in Year 10 classes at his local rural high school. Trent has been an outstanding student throughout his schooling, and his mother and father, a music teacher and lawyer, respectively, have high expectations of him. These include ongoing exemplary school grades leading to entry into a prestigious university course in the nearest city.

However, over the past few months, Trent's parents have noticed a distinct change in him. He is no longer interested in spending time with friends. His grades have slipped at school, and he appears dishevelled and distracted. Trent now prefers to spend his time alone in his messy room.

Attempts to raise their concerns have failed, as Trent refuses to talk to either the school counsellor or his parents. When at home he slinks off to his room to get away from their probing questions and worried expressions; his parents aren't quite sure if they should be more anxious, putting the behavioural changes down to adolescence. Still, his mother feels it could be something much more serious – a mental health problem – but she is reluctant to take her concerns outside the family environment. Her main concern is the stigma attached to mental illness, which she fears could ruin Trent's future. Confidentiality within the small country township is another significant worry.

VIGNETTE

Contemporary models of care

Current policy directions

Mental illness impacts upon an estimated 3.2 million Australians in any 12-month period, with around 3% of the overall Australian population experiencing severe mental illness such as bipolar disorder, schizophrenia or major depression. These illnesses, though varying in severity, have a profound effect on the individual, their family and the community in which they live (National Advisory Council on Mental Health [NACMH], 2010). People who experience severe and persistent mental illness require an intensive, integrated and innovative approach to their health needs in order for them to achieve optimum quality of life. The ability to recognise and minimise the impact that mental illness can have on the individual, their families and communities is a crucial factor in achieving positive therapeutic outcomes and indicates the ability of the practitioner to work within a culturally responsive paradigm (NACMH, 2010; Indigenous Allied Health Australia, 2013).

The changes and reforms of the Australian mental health system in recent decades have in some part come about to reflect society's changing attitudes and beliefs about mental health or illness. The term mental illness is now being used to encompass both common disorders such as depression, anxiety and substance use disorders, and low-prevalence disorders such as psychotic and eating disorders (Australian Institute of Health and Welfare, 2013).

The World Health Organization (WHO) recommends that all mental health policies are founded by four guiding principles. They are:

1 **Equity**: mental health resources should be fairly distributed as needed across the population
2 **Effectiveness**: mental health services should be aimed at improving health outcomes
3 **Efficiency**: available resources should be distributed for maximum gains for society and the individuals who make them up
4 **Access**: individuals have the right to utilise mental health treatment that is not based on one's ability to pay (WHO, 2003).

Australia's national and state plans and policies around mental health reflect both the WHO commitment to mental health and the United Nations' (UN) *Principles for the protection of persons with mental illness and the improvement of mental health care* (as cited in Hungerford et al., 2012).

Since the 1990s, the Australian mental health system has evolved from a system where care provision for individuals with severe and persistent mental illness was primarily provided in large residential psychiatric hospitals to the current community-focused model of care provision. This evolution has allowed for the development and expansion of both private and public clinical mental health services with the support of primary care, within-community and home-based mental health services. Further, the expansion of the non-government sector in the provision of psychosocial rehabilitation, advocacy and support of community development has moved forward. The most recent national mental health policies have highlighted the need for collaboration and integration of mental health care that is aimed at meeting the holistic and complex needs of individuals with mental health issues (NACMH, 2010). This collaboration is focused around five main areas:

- homelessness – through supported housing and outreach services to the homeless
- employment and education
- substance abuse
- improvements in physical health, and
- improved service integration between Justice and/or emergency services (NACMH, 2010).

However, there is some evidence to support an even more flexible approach in identifying and helping individuals and families within rural areas as 'current models of mental health service delivery do not adequately capture the early help-seeking dynamics of young rural men and their families' (Wilson, Cruickshank & Lea, 2012, p. 167).

Current mental health service provision is varied, just as the individuals who engage in these services have a variety of needs. Services span the health continuum and range from hospital and residential care, hospital-based outpatient and community mental healthcare services to consultations with specialist mental health professionals and general practitioners (GPs) (NACMH, 2010). Within the Australian context, access to mental health services can be complicated by factors such as geography. It is widely recognised within Australia that people living in rural and remote areas have poorer access to specialist mental healthcare services than their metropolitan counterparts, and evidence suggests that people residing in these areas have a higher prevalence of mental illness compared with the general population. One glaring example of this is the Western Area Health Service in New South Wales, which geographically covers over 55% of the state, with many of the population in this health service residing up to 400 km away from the nearest mental health inpatient facility (NACMH, 2010). The logistical issues in service provision to these low-density populations have given way to innovative practices to enable access to mental health care. One such innovation to address these challenges is the *Mental Health Emergency Care – Rural Access Program*, which utilises technology to conduct real-time mental health assessment and consultation (NACMH, 2010).

Current service frameworks

The public health framework is the overarching approach within which health services, including mental health services, are provided. This is especially relevant for those residing in rural/remote locations. The goal of this framework is to prevent illness and disease, promote positive health practices and increase life expectancy.

Mrazek and Haggerty's (1994) 'Spectrum of Interventions' (as cited in NSW Department of Health, 2008, p. 4) is widely accepted, used and adapted as a framework for defining mental health interventions within Australia. It forms the foundation for continuing national, state and territory mental health promotion, prevention, implementation and practice and also encompasses early intervention, treatment and recovery approaches.

The following descriptions are defined as they relate to mental health service delivery:

- mental health promotion: actions taken to maximise mental health among individuals and entire populations
- prevention: an intervention that has occurred prior to the initial onset of a disorder/illness to prevent its development
- early intervention: interventions that target individuals who display the early signs and symptoms of a mental health issue or mental disorder, and people beginning or experiencing a first episode of mental disorder/illness
- treatment: inclusive of early intervention, including proactive case identification (in clinical settings or clinical outreach) and evidence-based treatments for diagnosed disorders
- continuing care: interventions for individuals whose disorders continue or recur
- relapse prevention: interventions in response to the early warning signs of recurring mental disorder for people who have already experienced a mental disorder/illness (Commonwealth Department of Health and Aged Care, 2000).

Consumer and carer participation within mental healthcare service delivery in Australia is becoming increasingly common and is supported by a growing evidence base. The consumer-centred care approach to mental healthcare provision has a variety of benefits, including consumer carer satisfaction and increased adherence and effectiveness of evidence-based treatment options. They encompass three main principles where the individual:

- is unique
- is an equal member of their therapeutic team
- determines their responses to their life challenges.

Common examples of consumer-centred care used within the Australian mental health context include:

- person-centred approaches
- strengths-based approaches
- tidal model, and
- recovery model (Hungerford et al., 2012, p. 22).

VIGNETTE CONTINUED

Trent's mother receives a phone call from his school year advisor to discuss Trent's lack of engagement in class and failing grades. As a result, Trent agrees to an appointment with the family GP to assess Trent's physical and mental wellbeing. During this appointment, Trent tells his doctor he feels sad all the time but for no particular reason. He describes losing interest in activities he used to enjoy and neglecting his schoolwork because he does

>> not see the point. During this visit, Trent's doctor rules out any medical reasons for him feeling this way and talks to Trent about other possibilities, such as his mental health. After discussion about further options, Trent chooses to attend headspace for a mental health assessment. Trent is diagnosed with moderate depression and, after much consideration between Trent, his doctor and his mental health nurse (MHN), he commences on an antidepressant and agrees to see a MHN on a regular basis for cognitive behavioural therapy to help change his negative thought patterns.

Useful website:

National practice standards for the mental health workforce 2013
http://www.health.gov.au/internet/publications/publishing.nsf/Content/mental-pubs-n-wkstd13-toc~mental-pubs-n-wkstd13-3

Nurses and midwives' roles in supporting the mentally ill in rural Australia

The mental health workforce within Australia, though interdisciplinary, is primarily made up of five health professions: nursing, occupational therapy, psychiatry, psychology and social work. These professional bodies, along with government and other stakeholders, have collaboratively developed practice standards to which all health professionals working in the field of mental health should aspire (Victorian Government Department of Health, 2013). These standards, listed below, outline the types of knowledge, skills and attitudes that health professionals should possess when working within mental health services; they are also relevant to those health professionals not working in mental health as they serve as a guiding philosophy for healthcare service delivery.

The key principles of the *National Practice Standards for the Mental Health Workforce 2013* require that mental health professionals:

- promote an optimal quality of life for and with people with mental illness
- deliver services with the aim of facilitating sustained recovery
- involve people using services in all decisions regarding their treatment, care and support and, as far as possible, the opportunity to choose their treatment and setting
- recognise the right of the person to have their nominated carer involved in all aspects of their care

- learn about and value the lived experience of people using services, and their family or carers
- recognise the role played by carers, as well as their capacity, needs and requirements, separate from those of the person receiving services
- recognise and support the rights of children and young people affected by a family member with a mental illness to appropriate information, care and protection
- support participation by people and their families and carers as an integral part of mental health service development, planning, delivery and evaluation
- tailor mental health treatment, care and support to meet the specific needs of the individual
- in delivering mental health treatment and support impose the least personal restriction on the rights and choices of people, taking into account their living situation, level of support within the community, and the needs of their family or carer
- are aware of and implement evidence-informed practices and quality improvement processes
- participate in professional development activities and reflect what they have learnt in practice (Victorian Government Department of Health, 2013, p. 9).

The role of a MHN within the Australian landscape is continually evolving. Mental health nursing broadly refers to the provision of nursing and/or midwifery care to those experiencing mental illness and includes all aspects of care within the spectrum of interventions for mental health problems and disorders (Meadows, Singh & Grigg, 2012). The Australian and New Zealand College of Mental Health Nurses (ANZCMHN) has a more specific definition and defines a MHN as 'a registered nurse who holds a recognised specialist qualification in mental health nursing' (ANZCMHN, 1996). In spite of the varying definitions of a MHN, it is reasonable to say that all nurses, regardless of their chosen specialty or locality, will come into contact with and care for individuals experiencing mental ill-health. This is especially relevant for nurses and midwives working within rural health services where specialist mental health services may be outreached from larger townships. Nurses and midwives working within rural Australia have broad and varied roles. They are uniquely positioned as frontline health professionals to be the first point of contact for many individuals who present for health care.

People with severe and persistent mental illness experience ill-health as a further complication, resulting in the mortality risk for these individuals being 2.5 times higher than the general Australian population (NACMH, 2010).

The rural nurse and/or midwife's roles within health services (inclusive of integrated health services) are now more likely to include provision of not only physical care but also basic mental health care under the framework of collaborative care practices. This makes rural nurses and midwives an integral element in the provision of collaborative mental health care (Mahnken, 2001).

Fast forward 18 months and Trent, with the help of his family and health professionals, is no longer taking antidepressant medication but continues to see his MHN on a regular basis and is aware of his relapse early-warning signs and triggers. He is in his last year of high school and doing well both academically and socially. With the help of his MHN, Trent has developed new ways of coping with stress and negative thoughts and feelings and now feels hopeful and positive about his future.

Useful websites:

Chronic Disease eLearning
http://www.acmhn.org/chronic-disease-elearning

Perinatal eLearning
http://www.acmhn.org/perinatal-elearning

e-hub online mental health programs
http://www.ehub.anu.edu.au/

A Contributing Life: The 2013 National Report Card on Mental Health and Suicide Prevention
http://www.mentalhealthcommission.gov.au/our-2013-report-card.aspx

Summary

In this chapter, we have discussed how:

- generalist rural nurses and midwives play a vital role in supporting the mental health needs of rural communities
- promotion, prevention and early intervention strategies provide an overarching framework
- a lifespan approach is important, as children, adolescents, youth, adults and older adults all have specific needs
- in many instances rural clinicians provide first-line care in primary healthcare, community care and acute care environments
- alternatively, they provide the conduit to referral pathways to other members of the interdisciplinary assessment and treatment team, often involving contemporary technologies such as telemedicine
- a range of models of care are available that are designed to accommodate individual needs and service availability and access
- it is important for all rural clinicians to be aware of the Mental Health Act in their state or territory.

Reflective questions

1 Consider the specific mental health needs of people from a lifespan approach.
2 What do the four WHO guiding principles (i.e. equity, effectiveness, efficiency, access) mean to you?
3 What are the major issues relating to child and adolescent mental health in Australia?
4 What is your role as a nurse/midwife in the provision of care to individuals who are mentally ill?
5 How could you ensure Aboriginal and Torres Strait Islander Australians receive culturally appropriate and safe care?
6 Can you identify the services in your local community or broader health service that you would contact to help you provide holistic mental health care to a health user?
7 What could you do to reduce the stigma associated with mental ill-health?

References

Australian Bureau of Statistics (ABS). (2007). *National Survey of Mental Health and Wellbeing: Summary of Results.* Retrieved March 24, 2014, from www.ausstats.abs. gov.au/Ausstats/subscriber.nsf/0/6AE6DA447F985FC2CA2574EA00122BD6/ $File/43260_2007.pdf

Australian Centre for Posttraumatic Mental Health, *beyondblue*, Australian Centre for Grief and Bereavement, & Australian Red Cross. (2011). *Looking after yourself and your family after a disaster.* Melbourne: Australian Centre for Posttraumatic Mental Health, *beyondblue*, Australian Centre for Grief and Bereavement, & Australian Red Cross.

Australian Institute of Health and Welfare. (2013). *Mental health services in brief 2013.* Cat. no. HSE 141. Canberra: AIHW. Retrieved October 28, 2013, from http://www.aihw.gov.au/publication-detail/?id=60129544726

Australian and New Zealand College of Mental Health Nurses (ANZCMHN). (1996). *Constitution.* Adelaide: Australian and New Zealand College of Mental Health Nurses.

Beaton, T., Mann, R. & Grigg, M. (2011). Future directions. In K. Edward, I. Mundro, A. Robins & A. Welch (Eds.), *Mental health nursing: Dimensions of praxis* (pp. 517–30). Melbourne: Oxford University Press.

beyondblue. (2013a). *Beyondblue guide to the management of depression in primary care: A guide for health professionals.* Melbourne: *beyondblue*.

——. (2013b). Understanding anxiety and depression [Pamphlet]. Melbourne: *beyondblue*.

Commonwealth Department of Health and Aged Care. (2000). *Promotion, prevention and early intervention for mental health – a monograph.* Canberra: Mental Health and Special Programs Branch, Commonwealth Department of Health and Aged Care.

Department of Health and Ageing. (2009). *Fourth national mental health plan – An agenda for collaborative government action in mental health 2009–2014.* Canberra: Commonwealth of Australia. Retrieved March 24, 2014, from http://www.health. gov.au/internet/main/publishing.nsf/Content/9A5A0E8BDFC55D3BCA257BF 0001C1B1C/$File/plan09v2.pdf

Eckermann, A., Dowd, T., Chong, E., Nixon, L., Gray, R. & Johnson, S. (2010). *Binan Goonj: Bridging cultures in Aboriginal health* (3rd ed.). Chatswood NSW: Churchill Livingstone Elsevier.

Elder, R., Evans, K. & Nizette, D. (2013). *Psychiatric and mental health nursing* (3rd ed.). Sydney: Mosby Elsevier.

Garlick, R. & Koch, S. (2011). The older adult and mental illness. In K. Edward, I. Mundro, A. Robins & A. Welch (Eds.), *Mental health nursing: Dimensions of praxis* (pp. 251–74). Melbourne: Oxford University Press.

Gaynor, N., Harder, K., Munro, I. & Robins, A. (2011). Diagnostic systems used in clinical assessment. In K. Edward, I. Mundro, A. Robins & A. Welch (Eds.), *Mental health nursing: Dimensions of praxis* (pp. 27–50). Melbourne: Oxford University Press.

Happell, B., Cowin, L., Roper, C., Lakeman, R. & Cox, L. (2013). *Introducing mental health nursing: A service user-oriented approach* (2nd ed.). Crows Nest NSW: Allen & Unwin.

Hungerford, C., Clancy, R., Hodgson, D., Jones, T., Harrison, A. & Hart, C. (2012). *Mental health care: An introduction for health professionals.* Milton, Qld: Wiley & Sons Australia.

Hunter, E., Gill, N. & Toombs, M. (2013). Mental health among Indigenous Australians. In R. Hampton & M. Toombs (Eds.), *Indigenous Australians and health: The wombat in the room.* Melbourne: Oxford University Press.

Indigenous Allied Health Australia. (2013). *Improving cultural responsiveness of health professionals through education reform.* Canberra: IAHA Secretariat.

Jorm, A., Allen, N., Morgan, A., Ryan, S. & Purcell, R. (2013). *A guide to what works for depression* (2nd ed.). Melbourne: beyondblue. Retrieved March 24, 2014, from www.bspg.com.au/dam/bsg/product?client=BEYONDBLUE&prodid=BL/055 6&type=file

Kneisl, C., Wilson, H. & Trigoboff, E. (2004). *Contemporary psychiatric–mental health nursing.* Upper Saddle River, NJ: Pearson Prentice Hall.

Mahnken, J. E. (2001). Rural nursing and health care reforms: Building a social model of health. *Rural and Remote Health,* 1(104) (Online).

Meadows, G., Singh, B. & Grigg, M. (2012). *Mental health in Australia* (2nd ed.). Melbourne: Oxford University Press.

Munro, S. & Baker, J. (2007). Surveying the attitudes of acute mental health nurses. *Journal of Psychiatric & Mental Health Nursing*, 14(2), 196–202.

National Advisory Council on Mental Health (NACMH). (2010). *Fitting together the pieces: Collaborative care models for adults with severe and persistent mental illness – Final Project Report*. Retrieved March 24, 2014, from http://www.health.gov.au/internet/main/publishing.nsf/Content/mental-pubs-f-colsev

NSW Department of Health. (2008). *NSW community mental health strategy 2007–2012: From prevention and early intervention to recovery*. Sydney: NSW Department of Health.

Pederson, D. (2005). *Psych notes: Clinical pocket guide*. Philadelphia: FA Davis.

Petrie, E. (2011). Promoting mental health. In K. Edward, I. Mundro, A. Robins & A. Welch (Eds.), *Mental health nursing: Dimensions of praxis* (pp. 51–65). Melbourne: Oxford University Press. Retrieved March 24, 2014, from: http://www.health.gov.au/internet/main/publishing.nsf/Content/0ABBFD239D790377CA257BF0001C6CBC/$File/colsev.pdf

Plakiotis, C. & O'Connor, D. (2012). Psychiatric disorders affecting the elderly in Australia. In G. Meadows, M. Grigg, J. Farhall, F. McDermott, E. Fossey & B. Singh (Eds.), *Mental health in Australia: Collaborative community practice* (3rd ed.). Melbourne: Oxford University Press.

Reavley, N., Allen, N., Jorm, A., Morgan, A. & Purcell, R. (2010). *A guide to what works for anxiety disorders*. Melbourne: beyondblue.

Victorian Government Department of Health. (2013). National Practice Standards for the Mental Health Workforce 2013. Melbourne: Victorian Government Department of Health. Retrieved from http://www.health.gov.au/internet/main/publishing.nsf/Content/5D7909E82304E6D2CA257C430004E877/$File/wkstd13.pdf

West, R., Usher, K., Thompson, G. & Spurgeon, D. (2011). Indigenous (Australian and New Zealand) and remote mental health. In K. Edward, I. Mundro, A. Robins & A. Welch (Eds.), *Mental health nursing: Dimensions of praxis* (pp. 398–408). Melbourne: Oxford University Press.

Wilson, R., Cruickshank, M. & Lea, J. (2012). Experiences of families who help young rural men with emergent mental health problems in a rural community in New South Wales, Australia. *Contemporary Nurse*, 42(2), 167–77.

World Health Organization (WHO). (2003). *Organization of services for mental health. Mental health policy and service guidance package*. Geneva: WHO. Retrieved March 24, 2014, from http://www.who.int/mental_health/policy/services/4_organisation%20services_WEB_07.pdf

WHO Collaborating Centre for Evidence in Mental Health Policy. (2004). *Management of mental disorders: Treatment protocol project*, Vol. 2 (4th ed.). Darlinghurst, NSW: WHO Collaborating Centre for Evidence in Mental Health Policy.

10 Conducting research in rural contexts

Ysanne Chapman and Karen Francis

Learning objectives On completion of this chapter, the reader will be able to:

- discuss various reasons for implementing research

- describe the research process

- identify methods for data generation and collection

- list strategies for dissemination of research findings

- discuss the implications of research for rural nursing practice.

Key words ● Research, methodology, methods, dissemination, rural nursing and midwifery

Chapter overview

It is fitting that a chapter of this book considers the place of research in rural nursing. Research in health disciplines potentiates quality in healthcare delivery and can introduce new and effective evidence-based practices, consider the success and usefulness of health policies, or describe and comment on clients' or patients' experiences of particular phenomena. Initiating research may at times seem an overwhelming venture, and we hope this chapter will provide some insights into how to start. The authors have used a research study they undertook in 2007 with three other colleagues on overseas trained nurses' experiences in rural settings as an exemplar to illustrate the approaches adopted to ask and answer questions of practice (Francis, Chapman, Doolan, Sellick & Barnett, 2008).

Introduction

Good research stems from a well-designed and articulated research proposal. The proposal is a snapshot that captures the depth and breadth of the research study and provides a frame of reference as researchers progress the research. Without a robust proposal, research can be fragmented, tangential or may never come to fruition. Initial ideas about a research project can be captured on a one-page document and diagram. This summary can be used to 'sell' the research idea to collaborators and provide a template to develop a proposal (see Figure 10.1).

A good research proposal can be reused in dissemination of the research, in providing succinct information to ethics committees or with a view to attracting others to the research team. Research proposals are needed for all research projects, and the framework suggested here can be adapted for either higher degree study or commissioned research. The structure adopted for this chapter contains the necessary requirements for any research proposal.

Research title

Every piece of written work requires a title, and research proposals are no exception. Research titles should not be obscure or ethereal – rather, they should express the substantive nature of the research. A research title should be tight, simple and clear. An example of a clear research title is: 'Using overseas registered nurses to fill employment gaps in rural health services: Quick fix or sustainable strategy?' (Francis et al., 2008). This research title identifies the focus, the people involved and the intention of the research. It uses plain language and adheres to MeSH terms (see below).

Conversely, an example of an unclear research title is: 'The horse on the dining room table'. This title is a colloquialism that is culturally bound and not recognised by people outside that culture. The title as it stands is not inclusive of MeSH or other codes used to describe areas of research. This title could be used with additional information clarifying the research intent: 'The horse on the dining room table: Exploring dying and death in residential aged care – a grounded theory'. The revised title now heralds the intent of the investigation and provides a glimpse of the research design and the research context while

Overseas registered nurses in rural hospitals
Research by Francis, Chapman, Doolan, Selleck & Barnett

Why?
What is the experience of the Gippsland rural health agencies in recruiting and retaining overseas nurses who have been trained in non-traditional countries?
Can a best practice model of recruitment and retention be devised for use by rural health agencies in the Gippsland region?

Subquestions:
- What methods are used to recruit overseas nurses from non-traditional countries?
- What is the experience of overseas nurses from non-traditional countries who have been recruited to rural practice?
- What is the experience of employers of overseas nurses from non-traditional countries who have been recruited to rural practice?
- What are considered successful strategies for what? What are the barriers?

What?
Areas for further investigation:
- Recruitment strategies
- Retention strategies – 'fit' for practice, 'fit' for environment
- Family incentives
- Costs to the nurses themselves – fiscal and emotional
- Costs to the employer – fiscal

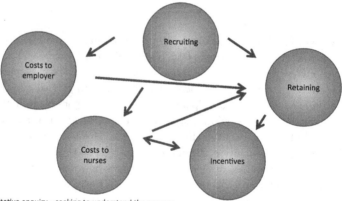

How?
- Qualitative enquiry – seeking to understand the process

Who?
- Named researchers
- Rural hospitals in Victoria
  - Employers
  - Peers
  - Nurses themselves

Funding?
- Internal research grant – university
- State Health Department – recruitment and retention planning
- Nurses Board of Victoria incentive grants

FIGURE
10.1

Ideas for research with overseas registered nurses.

keeping an artistic element to capture the readers' interest. For consistency, the exemplar – 'Using overseas registered nurses to fill employment gaps in rural health services: Quick fix or sustainable strategy?' – will be used throughout this chapter to illustrate the various dimensions of constructing a research proposal.

Abstract

This summary of the research should provide the reader with sufficient information about the substantive nature and methodological prowess of the research. Usually abstracts are 250–300 words in length and couched in layman's language. Abstracts tend to whet the appetite of the readers and therefore should be somewhat 'punchy'. They need to 'grab' the attention of the readers and detail enough information for them to make decisions about the value and congruency of the research. Using our earlier exemplar, the abstract is detailed below (Figure 10.2).

Objective: This study sought to identify and evaluate approaches used to attract internationally trained nurses from traditional and non-traditional countries and incentives employed to retain them in small rural hospitals in Gippsland, Victoria. **Design**: An exploratory descriptive design. **Setting**: Small rural hospitals in Gippsland, Victoria. **Participants**: Hospital staff responsible for recruitment of nurses and overseas trained nurses from traditional and non-traditional sources (e.g. England, Scotland, India, Zimbabwe, Holland, Singapore, Malaysia). **Results and Conclusion**: Recruitment of married overseas trained nurses is more sustainable than that of single registered nurses; however, the process of recruitment for the hospital and potential employees is costly. Rural hospitality diffuses some of these expenses by means of the employing hospitals providing emergency accommodation and necessary furnishings. Cultural differences and dissonance regarding practice create barriers for some of the overseas trained nurses to move towards a more sanguine position. On the positive side, single overseas registered nurses use the opportunity to work in rural Australian hospitals as an effective working holiday that promotes employment in larger, more specialised hospitals. Overall, both the registered nurses and the employees believe the experience to be beneficial rather than detrimental.

FIGURE 10.2 *Sample abstract related to research study exemplar (Adapted from Francis et al., 2008, p. 164).*

Key words

Key words actually identify the main areas of focus of the research. They are codes that highlight the fields of research and enhance abilities to link like-minded research topics and genres. There are several lists of key words that are acceptable in labelling research; for example, MeSH, FoR and SEO provide links to internet sites. Figure 10.3 below lists the key words utilised for our chosen exemplar.

Overseas registered nurse

Recruitment

Retention

Rural

FIGURE
10.3 *Example of key words for research study exemplar.*

The call to the question

Researchers are brought to research activity for a number of reasons. Some of these include extensions of research performed earlier, personal or professional insights into problems that can be researched, a need to test the success of an intervention, or a nagging doubt about a particular issue. Whatever the impetus for the research, the reasons should be declared. For example, the impetus to investigate overseas registered nurses arose from growing usage of these nurses to staff rural hospitals and also concerns that support systems were not well established to accommodate their unique needs. These issues were being debated in many policy forums and by regulatory authorities that were redeveloping licensure requirements for internationally qualified nurses seeking employment in Australia (Kingma, 2001; Walker, 2008; Deegan & Simkin, 2010; Dean, 2011).

Background to the study (literature review)

Literature reviews can be contentious issues. Some methodologies demand rigorous literature reviews; others suggest that looking at the literature may potentiate some bias when embarking on analysis. It is important to be very familiar with the position related to literature reviews using the methodology of choice in your study. Having an intimate knowledge of the methodology adopted for the study guides decisions regarding structure of the background or literature review to the study. The background to the study should articulate what is known on the topic of interest and what the knowledge deficits are, and it should substantiate the need to undertake the study. Phenomenologists, for example, develop a discussion of related issues that inform understanding but do not conduct a review of literature directly related to the research question – they assert that a literature review per se will add to their prior knowledge of the phenomenon and potentially limits the analysis process, retarding the researcher's ability to see the text for itself (McConnell-Henry, Chapman & Francis, 2009).

Undertaking a literature review involves organising a process to search the literature. What is needed is a strategy to locate and retrieve the pertinent information, decisions on inclusion and exclusion criteria, the use of a specific time frame to further limit the literature gathered, and stipulation of a language in which the papers/data source are published.

There is a growing trend for researchers to conduct what they refer to as a systematic review of the literature. This process, like a literature review, is a systematic method for isolating quality research directly related to their research topics. Appraising the quality of research is achieved using standardised criteria. Quantitative researchers report on the validity of the research, which is the '... extent to which the findings of a study accurately reflect the phenomena being measured' and the reliability that '... relates to the ability of a research design to consistently reflect a phenomenon over time' (Nagy, Mills, Waters & Birks, 2010, p. 179). Qualitative researchers appraise research for its trustworthiness. This is achieved by assessing the credibility, fittingness, auditability and confirmability of the research approach, data generation analysis techniques and the presented findings (Nagy et al., 2010).

Undertaking a systematic review requires details of the search strategy used to locate research and other data sources including, but not limited to, reports, policy documents and diaries that inform understanding of the topic and/or phenomenon of interest to be stated. The search strategy details inclusion criteria: the type of publications that will be included, such as research papers that are assessed using tools to rank research rigour (Richardson-Tench, Taylor, Kermode & Roberts, 2011). Being clear about how the literature is sourced and articulating the decision trail that has been used to guide this process add to the overall quality of the proposal.

The literature review undertaken in our exemplar isolated what was known about the topic and highlighted the knowledge gaps and gave credence to our study initiatives.

The research question

Isolating the research question is achieved when the topic is understood. The topic is the global idea that has piqued the researcher's interest. For example, there may be interest in how children cope with a chronic illness. From this topic of global interest, a research question is developed that allows the phenomenon, children coping with a chronic illness, to be investigated. Seasoned researchers turn to the research questions to see if they reflect congruence between methodo-logy and method. The research question in this context is not necessarily the question asked of the participants involved in the research study; rather, it is the hypothesis (true or null) to be proven or the substantive focus of the study. The overall research question frames what it is the researchers want to know.

In our study with overseas registered nurses, the research questions were:

- What is the experience of the Gippsland rural health agencies in recruiting and retaining overseas nurses who have been trained in non-traditional countries?
- Can a best practice model of recruitment and retention be devised for use by rural health agencies in the Gippsland region?

Methodology

Methodology is not method; rather, it is the philosophical framework, the worldview or paradigm from which the approach has evolved. Worldviews refer to an individual or society's belief systems, values, ideas and ethics that underpin how the world is interpreted and interacted with. A worldview or paradigm encompasses assumptions about:

> ...what is real, what is true, what is acceptable, what and who are most powerful, and even the very nature of people, objects, and events in the world (McMurray, Pace & Scott, 2004, p. 9).

Positivists (quantitative research traditions align with this worldview), for example, propose that knowledge is based on logical inference that is derived from data generated through sensory experience, and that is analysed and verified using logical and mathematical treatments. This worldview subscribes to a belief that individuals and societies are predictable; this tradition is epistemological – that is, a theory of knowledge. Researchers using a quantitative methodology seek definitive answers, a singular truth that can be generalised. Research questions posed are linked to analytical deductive statements that explain and can be tested to determine a singular truth that explains the phenomenon of interest. This methodological tradition or worldview is reductionist in nature (Stumpf & Fieser, 2003) – that is, what is observed can be explained without qualification.

Qualitative research methodologies, on the other hand, are generally described as belonging to the interpretivist, or critical, paradigm or worldview. These worldviews hold that living is complex and that individuals experience the world differently. There is not a singular truth to explain and predict; rather, multiple truths are accepted and justified. Interpretivist research methodologies are characteristically inductive investigations that seek to illuminate what it is to be human. Interpretivism is therefore both epistemological (i.e. knowledge generating) and ontological (the study of being and existing in the world). Qualitative researchers do not seek to pose questions that will lead to generalisations but rather to increase understanding of the complexity of humanity, thus accommodating difference. It is this very aspect of this worldview that is often cited as a key criticism of interpretivist approaches (Denzin & Lincoln, 2003; Taylor, Kermode & Roberts, 2006). The refinement of a research question/s should therefore inform the choice of methodology utilised.

Our study with overseas registered nurses was qualitative in nature. It aimed to understand the processes involved in the recruitment and retention of these nurses in rural hospitals. This study was largely explorative and used a critical ethnographic philosophical intent, which in turn informed the methods utilised. Ethical approval to conduct the study was sought from our employing university's Human Ethics Committee. As required, our research project adhered to the principles of the National Health and Medical Research Council (NHMRC) for conducting ethical human research (NHMRC, 2007).

Methods

This is the 'how to' of a research proposal: recruitment of participants, and how data are collected, stored and ultimately analysed. In this section, the researcher needs to maintain congruence between the research question, the research methodology and the methods.

Recruitment of participants

Recruitment of participants generally commences as soon as ethics approval is obtained. Participants are recruited according to certain criteria that describe the characteristics of the types of participants needed. For example, these may include age, gender, occupation, English speaking, having experienced a phenomenon of interest such as migrating to Australia, and a willingness to be involved. Participants may be recruited using a variety of methods such as advertising in local, national and international newspapers, radio or television, flyers displayed in strategic settings such as a workplace, and online recruitment using social media. Researchers are not permitted under the NHMRC guidelines to directly recruit; an intermediary person or process must be used. For our study, we placed flyers in wards of targeted hospitals describing the study and providing information about how potential participants could contact us. Interested persons contacted us by either telephone or post. After hearing from interested persons, we contacted them to give additional information as required and to establish recruitment.

Collection of data

The techniques adopted for the collection of data must align with the chosen methodology. Phenomenological researchers usually generate data through one-to-one interviews with participants, while action researchers are likely to work with groups and use group processes such as focus groups, Delphi techniques and small group work to collect data. Historians may use these techniques coupled with collecting artifacts that were used, built or produced and documentation such as official records, personal diaries, newspapers or posters produced during the period of time under investigation (Francis, 2013a; Sweeney, 2005). Researchers using discourse analysis methodology may source data from reports, documents and grey literature in a similar manner to that of historians.

Management of data

How are data managed? That is, what are the processes adopted by researchers to organise the data for the purpose of analysis (understanding)? Raw data can take the following forms: oral conversations; written texts such as diary entries, reports or policy statements; paintings; buildings; or other artifacts that provide insights into people's lives. Conversational data are transformed to text through transcription of interviews or focus group conversations prior to analysis. Other non-textual data – such as artwork, music and domestic implements – are often considered in conjunction with reference to other textual data sources such as expert opinion, historical essays, diaries, government reports and so on. Non-textual data are interpreted and thus explained in text; for example, photo-elicitation (Bignante, 2010). Typically, a global review of the data to establish overall content understanding is performed. Next, data (text) are sorted using a pre-devised plan, which can be as simple as searching the text for significant themes or strings of words that have resonance; alternatively, in some cases, a template is used that may be modelled on categories or codes that were identified in the initial review of the data. Researchers crosscheck the categories; they modify and synthesise them as necessary until they reach a point at which they are able to explain the meaning of the full data set, drawing on the known body of knowledge to justify their interpretations. Using a template that provides a visual representation of the relationship between text or artifact and theme or code development is a useful technique. Data management programs such as NVivo, Ethnograph or even Excel that can be used to categorise data sets are available to help researchers manage data. A word processing program is a primary tool of contemporary researchers, and for some it is the only computer program required.

Analysis of data

Making sense of the data is the stage of the research process often referred to as the analysis phase. Generation of global statements that explain the essence of the text or other data as it relates to the research question/s posed is a common approach. Key to this process is aligning the analysis with the intent of the research. Rigour is established in this process when the researcher is able to describe how these statements were developed and why, and by providing evidence links to the text as exemplars. Researchers exploring messages within textual documentation – such as those using a discourse analysis methodology

(Francis, 2013b) – will ask the text questions such as who is speaking and why, who has given permission for them to speak as a process for interrogating the text, and uncovering covert and overt power relationships that direct societal and individual behaviours.

Using the exemplar of our study with overseas registered nurses, we gathered data using interviews from key informants (the nurses themselves and the employers in rural hospitals). Analysis of the interview data was undertaken by asking key questions: Who said this? For what reasons? Was there any gain to be had? Who was silenced in this discourse, and why?

Significance of the study (the 'so what?' question)

Investing in research is a time-consuming process that ultimately needs justification. Questions that emanate from the researchers, funding agencies and consumers of the research may be: Why do the study? What are the possible implications of doing the study? Justifying outcomes can be fraught with challenges, particularly when the study is small-scale and addresses questions that are not world-shattering or life-threatening. Qualitative researchers undertake research that is about human existence (like our study about the plight of overseas registered nurses) and, while some studies will have a significant impact and resonate with many people, other studies will be less dramatic. Making a difference through generating understanding of humanity is the penultimate outcome of any qualitative research inquiry. Relating the findings to the body of knowledge and highlighting the gap in this knowledge addressed by the study is a highly credible outcome. Further, reflecting on the implications for practice and policy and making recommendations for change impact positively on populations.

Possible outcomes

The impetus for undertaking any research study is to generate knowledge. The knowledge generated from research studies may have a global impact, such as the refinement of in vitro fertilisation methods to enhance human fertility (Monash IVF, 2012) or the development of new drugs such as fingolimod to delay the progression of multiple sclerosis and decrease relapse (Multiple Sclerosis Trust, 2012). Many research endeavours, however, have less sensational outcomes, and yet they make a significant contribution that adds to knowledge. For example, an Australian study undertaken by Adams et al. (2012) to promote healthy eating in urban Aboriginal people in Geelong, Victoria, raised participants' awareness about food security and advocated working with Aboriginal communities using culturally appropriate methods to promote healthy eating. Another study that utilised a discourse analysis methodology to examine maternity care policy in Australia illustrated how policy can be influenced by stakeholders (McIntyre, Francis & Chapman, 2012). Each of the examples provided demonstrates a contribution to knowledge and highlights the diversity of impact that research studies can have. Our exemplar study informed the policy, process of recruitment and retention at a local level where the study was conducted.

Timelines

Conceptualising a research study and planning the process of completing the study must include consideration of timelines. Researchers need to identify realistic timelines that detail the beginning and the end point, or when the study will be completed. The timeline can be developed as a series of tasks, with dates for each task or set of tasks to be finalised by (see Figure 10.4).

ACTIVITY/MONTH	MARCH	APR–SEPT	OCT	NOV	DEC
Develop instrument	X				
Prepare and submit ethics application	X				
Obtain ethics approval		X			
Recruit participants		X			
Study intervention period		X			
Data collection		X	X		
Data analysis			X		
Prep of final report and pubs				X	X

FIGURE 10.4 *An example of a simple research timeline.*

Researchers will often utilise a Gantt chart as a tool to capture the timeline established (see Figure 10.5).

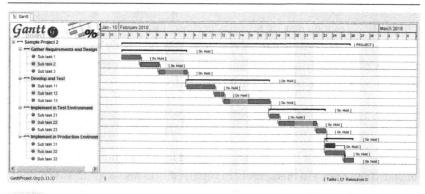

FIGURE 10.5 *Project management Gantt chart template (Project Remedies Inc., 2012).*

Dissemination

As previously indicated, research should inform understanding. For knowledge to be supplemented by research, it is imperative that research is shared. Dissemination of research can occur through writing reports, posting information on websites, presenting at conferences, publishing in peer-reviewed journals (as with our exemplar study), media interviews (television, radio and newspaper) and publications. Research can also be disseminated through conversations with individuals, groups, communities and key stakeholders that may include government or, in the case of commercially marketable research outcomes (e.g. patents for new technologies or drugs), investors willing to pay for the rights to reproduce these outcomes for profit.

Budget

Developing a budget that details the costs for conducting a research study is necessary if funding is to be sought. Budgets typically include four broad areas of support: personnel, equipment, travel and other.

Personnel

In this section of a budget, researcher time may be included as a budget item if the funding body supports payment for this item. Administrative support and other specialist assistance such as a transcriber, statistician, graphic designer, information technologist or research personnel are included in this budget line. Costings for personnel may be calculated on an hourly basis or on a daily, monthly or yearly basis. Depending on the instructions provided by targeted funding bodies, on-costs may also be included.

Equipment

Equipment that must be purchased or rented for completion of the research is included and costed in this section. Equipment includes such items as computers, digital voice recorders, iPads, data management/analysis software and specialised technology that may include microscopes, animals for experimentation and so on. Quotations for the purchase of requested items should be sought, ensuring that the budget reflects actual costs. In addition, costs associated with communication systems, printing, laboratory supplies and such like must also provide quotations.

Travel

Many research projects involve researcher travel, travel of specialists recruited to support the project, or travel of participants who have agreed to be involved. Obtaining quotations for air, train or bus travel is common and calculating car travel expenses normally uses a criterion adopted by the funding body (government or private industry). In this section, meal allowances may also be included.

Other

Any additional items that cannot be included in the other sections are listed here. Infrastructure costs and levies imposed by organisations for use of their facilities are often included in this section. The following web links provide useful information on how to construct a research project budget:

http://www.washington.edu/research/?page=budgetdevelopment
http://www.uaa.alaska.edu/research/OSP/budget-preparation.cfm

A justification of each budget item should be included detailing what the roles of the personnel will be, and each of the other items must be explicated.

Holly is a registered nurse who works in a rural general practice. She has responsibility for conducting childhood immunisations (under the supervision of the general practitioner) and preschool checks. The population that accesses this general practice includes local Indigenous families, Sudanese and Zimbabwean refugees, non-Indigenous Australian families of various socioeconomic disadvantage, and a small proportion of families from each group who do not believe in immunisation of their children.

VIGNETTE

In the community where Holly works, there has been a significant rise in the outbreak of pertussis (whooping cough). She believes that the community may have become complacent about immunisation of children and feels that it is timely to raise awareness of childhood immunisation benefits.

Questions
1 How might Holly achieve her outcome?
2 How would Holly know if her strategies have been successful?
3 How might Holly inform other health service providers and policy makers of her performance?

Summary

In this chapter, we have:

- provided direction for undertaking a research project
- outlined each step of the research process and given examples
- emphasised the importance of research in rural nursing practice
- whet the reader's appetite for engaging in research.

Reflective questions

1 Describe the research process.
2 Identify a topic of interest and craft a research question that will enable investigation.
3 Discuss how this research will impact on nursing practice.
4 What data will need to be generated to answer question 2? (Note: make sure there is congruence between the research question and the methods employed to answer the question.)
5 List ways in which the data might be managed.
6 List at least four avenues for dissemination of this research.

References

Adams, K., Burns, C., Liebzeit, A., Ryschka, J., Thorpe, S. & Browne, J. (2012). Use of participatory research and photo-voice to support urban Aboriginal healthy eating. *Health and Social Care in the Community*, 20(5), 497–505. doi: 10.1111/j.1365–2524.2011.01056.x

Bignante, E. (2010). The use of photo-elicitation in field research. *Echo-Geo*, 11. Retrieved March 24, 2014, from http://echogeo.revues.org/11466

Dean, E. (2011). Patient safety marred by lack of clarity over English skills testing. *Nursing Standard*, 25(29), 5.

Deegan, J. & Simkin, K. (2010). Expert to novice: Experiences of professional adaptation reported by non-English speaking nurses in Australia. *Australian Journal of Advanced Nursing*, 27(3), 31–7.

Denzin, N. K. & Lincoln, Y. S. (2003). Introduction: The discipline and practice of qualitative research. In N. K. Denzin & Y. S. Lincoln (Eds.) *The landscape of qualitative research: Theories and issues* (2nd ed.). Thousand Oaks, Calif: Sage.

Francis, K. (2013a). Historical research. In B. Taylor & K. Francis. *Qualitative research in health sciences: Methodologies, methods and processes* (pp. 56–65). Milton Park, Oxon, UK: Routledge.

——. (2013b). Discourse analysis. In B. Taylor & K. Francis. *Qualitative research in health sciences: Methodologies, methods and processes* (pp. 258–65). Milton Park, Oxon, UK: Routledge.

Francis, K., Chapman, Y., Doolan, G., Sellick, K. & Barnett, T. (2008). Using overseas registered nurses to fill employment gaps in rural health services: Quick fix or sustainable strategy? *Australian Journal of Rural Health*, 16(3), 164–9. doi: 10.1111/j.1440–1584.2008.00967.x

Kingma, M. (2001). Nursing migration: Global treasure hunt or disaster-in-the-making? *Nursing Inquiry*, 8(4), 205–12. doi: 10.1046/j.1440–1800.2001.00116.x

McConnell-Henry, T., Chapman, Y. & Francis, K. (2009). Husserl and Heidegger: Exploring the disparity. *International Journal of Nursing Practice*, 15(1), 7–15. doi: 10.1111/j.1440–172X.2008.01724.x

McIntyre, M., Francis, K. & Chapman, Y. (2012). Critical discourse analysis: Understanding change in maternity services. *International Journal of Nursing Practice*, 18(1), 36–43. doi: 10.1111/j.1440–172X.2011.01991.x

McMurray, A. J., Pace, R. W. & Scott, D. (2004). *Research: A commonsense approach*. Sth Melbourne, Vic: Thomson.

Monash IVF. (2012). *Life starts here*. Melbourne: Healthbridge Hawthorn Private Hospital. Retrieved March 24, 2014, from http://www.monashivf.com

Multiple Sclerosis Trust. (2012). Fingolimod (Gilenya) [Factsheet]. Retrieved March 24, 2014, from http://www.mstrust.org.uk/information/publications/factsheets/fingolimod.jsp

Nagy, S., Mills, J., Waters, D. & Birks, M. (2010). *Using research in healthcare practice*. Broadway: Wolters Kluwer, Lippincott, Williams & Wilkins.

National Health & Medical Research Council of Australia (NHMRC). (2007). *National Statement on Ethical Conduct in Human Research*. Canberra: Australian Government. Retrieved March 24, 2014, from http://www.nhmrc.gov.au/_files_nhmrc/publications/attachments/e72.pdf

Project Remedies Inc. (2012). *Project portfolio management consulting and solutions.* Pittsburgh, PA: Project Management Inc. Retrieved March 24, 2014, from http://www.projectremedies.com/software-products.php

Richardson-Tench, M., Taylor, B., Kermode, S. & Roberts, K. (2011). *Research in nursing: Evidence for best practice* (4th ed.). Sth Melbourne, Vic: Cengage Learning Australia.

Stumpf, S. E. & Fieser, J. (2003). *Philosophy: History and problems* (6th ed.). Boston: McGraw Hill.

Sweeney, J. F. (2005). Historical research: Examining documentary sources. *Nurse Researcher,* 12(3), 61–73.

Taylor, B., Kermode, S. & Roberts, K. (2006). *Research in nursing and health care: Evidence for practice* (3rd ed.). Sth Melbourne, Vic: Thomson.

Walker, L. (2008). A mixed picture: The experiences of overseas trained nurses in New Zealand. *Kai Tiaki Nursing New Zealand,* 14(11), 18–19.

11 Conclusion

SUSTAINING THE HEALTH OF RURAL POPULATIONS

Karen Francis, Ysanne Chapman, Faye McMillan and Jane Havelka

Learning objectives

On completion of this chapter, the reader will be able to:

- discuss the implications for nursing practice in rural and remote Australia
- describe the diversity of populations who reside in rural and remote Australia
- appreciate the common health challenges of rural people at each stage of the lifespan
- identify strategies for securing a sustainable nursing and midwifery workforce for rural and remote practice
- isolate future opportunities for nurses and midwives working in rural and remote practice settings.

Key words

- Rural and remote populations, culture, health status, nursing and midwifery, research

Chapter overview

The final chapter provides a précis of the book content followed by concluding remarks on the future of rural communities, the health workforce, and challenges and opportunities for nurses and midwives who wish to practise and advance their careers in rural settings.

Introduction

Understanding the nature and character of rural Australia and of the people who live there is a prerequisite for anyone contemplating practice in these contexts. The vastness of the land and the diversity of the populations who reside in it are reflective of the opportunities available. Nurses and midwives are the largest group of health professionals and the most evenly distributed throughout

Australia (Francis & Mills, 2011; Health Workforce Australia [HWA], 2012). The contribution they make to the health and wellbeing of rural Australians is significant. Choosing to work in rural and remote Australia is a wise career option that affords opportunities to extend and advance practice that impacts positively on individuals, groups and communities.

The challenge for health professionals is staying motivated to celebrate the diversity of rural Australia (and in fact all of Australia) and to find innovative ways to be culturally responsive. The accountability for delivering culturally responsive health care is on individual health professionals to appropriately respond to the unique cultural attributes of the person, family or community with whom they are working. Using a culturally responsive framework creates an environment that empowers all parties in the relationship and seeks to provide opportunities that recognise the whole individual and contributions that produce an action (see Figure 11.1). The notion of cultural responsiveness means that health professionals can apply this principle to all facets of health service delivery and respect the uniqueness and diversity of the communities in which they work (Indigenous Allied Health Australia [IAHA], 2013).

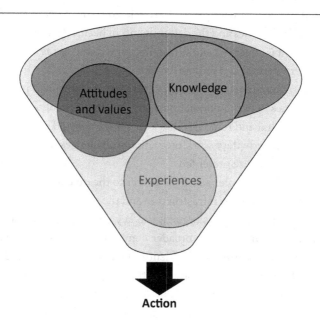

FIGURE 11.1   *Concept of cultural responsiveness – represented visually (IAHA, 2013).*

Summary of content

This text was designed to introduce readers to rural and remote Australia and provide direction for working in the range of practice contexts available. The authors who have contributed are predominantly experienced registered nurses and/or midwives, whilst others are registered health professionals; they all have experience of working in rural and remote Australia. In addition, two of the authors are Aboriginal women from rural areas. All agree that being prepared for both the challenges and rewards facilitates a successful transition to practice.

The first section of the text provides initial information on rural and remote Australia and highlights features of the health workforce employed in these settings. **Chapter 1** introduces readers to the diversity of the Australian population, highlighting the colourful history of the nation and the contribution of Indigenous peoples and the successive waves of immigrants who have contributed to the evolution of a unique 'Australian' culture. The variable weather conditions and geography of the continent are described, and the implications for government particularly related to health care are discussed. National health priorities and the determinants of health feature in this chapter, and an argument is advanced situating nurses and midwives as central to health service delivery in rural and remote locations.

Classification systems used to define 'rurality' are explained in **Chapter 2.** Health disparities between populations who live in metropolitan communities compared with rural and remote settings are portrayed, and an overview of the rural nursing and midwifery workforce and the challenges these clinicians face in the delivery of care are presented.

Chapter 3. This chapter alerts the reader to the diversity of rural communities in terms of resources, infrastructure and the peoples who reside in them. Knowing the community, it is argued, is a key strategy for facilitating access by individuals, groups and the broader community to resources that enable the achievement of 'health for all'. Identifying healthcare needs and developing methods for meeting these feature in this chapter. Supporting community members to traverse the healthcare system is advocated and predicated on health professionals (including nurses and midwives) having a sound knowledge of local services and those that can be accessed from – or at – a distance.

Chapter 4 examines in detail rural nursing and midwifery. As the largest group of health professionals, nurses are integral providers of health in all contexts of practice. In rural and remote settings they are the mainstay of health care. Likewise, the work of midwives is essential for the continuation of accessible maternity care in rural and remote settings. Working in rural and remote settings is both challenging and rewarding, requiring knowledge and practice wisdom specific to the context of practice. Being prepared and understanding how to harness the resources at hand are integral to success.

The second section of the text looks at the population using a lifespan approach, delineating the specific needs of age groups and the roles that rural nurses and midwives have in meeting these.

Chapter 5 is dedicated to examining reproductive health. Pregnancy as a normal life event is explored. Nurses and midwives' roles in supporting women are featured, with particular emphasis on birthing women. Paternity is discussed in terms of a role that many men, including those who reside in rural and remote settings, experience.

Chapter 6. Growing up in rural Australia is both an advantage and a disadvantage. Health prevention practices – including childhood immunisation programs – are described, and common illnesses and injuries impacting on children are discussed.

Chapter 7. Adulthood in rural communities covers employment opportunities and the impact that these have on health and wellbeing. Common health concerns and preventative healthcare initiatives to promote wellbeing are featured.

Chapter 8. Ageing is a normal life event. Living in a rural community and being an ageing person is the focus of this chapter. The promotion of self-care as a strategy for living longer and living well in this context is highlighted using a case study approach. Harnessing resources available in the community to support ageing is a feature of the case study.

Chapter 9. Using a lifespan approach, an overview of mental health and wellbeing in rural communities is presented in this chapter. The specific needs of Aboriginal and Torres Strait Islander people who reside in these settings are discussed. Contemporary models of health care utilised by nurses and midwives and other members of the multidisciplinary healthcare team are covered.

Chapter 10. Using evidence to underpin practice is an expectation of all nurses and midwives. The competency standards that direct practice of both nurses and midwives reinforce this mandate (Nurses and Midwives Accreditation Council, 2012). Appreciating the value of research, contributing to the research agenda and using research in practice are topics covered in this chapter. The chapter provides a guide for doing research and explores options for sharing research outcomes so that the nursing, midwifery and broader health knowledge base is expanded.

The future of rural communities

Rural communities are changing as the economy of the nation is in a transition phase. Traditional businesses are being challenged as online retail options provide people with easy access to greater diversity of goods at lower prices (Keane, 2013; KPMG, 2013). Keane warns that if businesses fail to recognise the impact that technology is having on the retail sector, they will become obsolete (2013). For many rural inhabitants, the loss of retail from their communities has and will continue to have a significant impact on employment and therefore attractiveness to current and potential residents. The incidence of mental health disorders such as anxiety and depression, and rising suicide rates among men specifically, is of concern. Rural communities that are experiencing decline are often characterised by older population demographics. Loneliness and living in poverty are two features of aged populations that have been linked to rising incidences of anxiety and depression.

These morbidity and mortality trends for older rural men aged 45 and above are largely linked to economic downturn (*beyondblue*, 2013; National Rural Health Alliance [NRHA], 2009). Suicide rates among younger rural men (aged 15–44 years) are twice as high as those of metropolitan counterparts because of unemployment, access to harmful weapons, alcohol and drug misuse, loneliness and relationship breakdown (NRHA, 2009). Indigenous rural men are six times more likely to commit suicide than those who reside in metropolitan communities. These data are alarming and have warranted attention leading to the development of a national suicide prevention strategy (Australian Government, 2012). Further, a number of government and non-government organisations offer programs and support to vulnerable groups such as youth, rural populations and older adults – for example, ReachOut (ReachOut, 2013), Communities Matter (Suicide Prevention Australia, 2013) and *beyondblue* (*beyondblue*, 2013). The impact of the current global financial crisis continues to be felt by many Australians. While Australia is an affluent nation by world standards, there are still many who live in poverty and have poorer life chances than others. A focus on addressing such inequity will continue to be a feature of the Australian Government's policies, and of health specifically. Raising health literacy is one strategy that must continue to feature as part of the overall health targets of government and healthcare services.

While many rural communities have declined, there are also those who have prospered. The mining industry boom discussed in Chapter 7 has led to significant population changes and an associated growth in building, recreational, transportation, education and health sector development.

Rural health workforce

There is no doubt that nurses will continue to be the largest group of health professionals in the Australian health workforce, and specifically in the rural and remote health workforce (HWA, 2012). Unlike other health professionals, nurses and midwives are relatively evenly distributed in all contexts of practice and therefore make a significant contribution to communities' access to health care and overall population health. Health Workforce Australia (Banks, 2005; HWA, 2011), and prior to them the Health Productivity Commission report (Banks, 2005), signalled that nurses were invaluable and that advancing their practice was a strategic approach to improve health outcomes particularly for vulnerable populations, including rural and remote peoples. Advanced practice nurses who include, but are not limited to, nurse practitioners have become a common feature of the health landscape. Expanded practice for many nurses and midwives includes prescribing, referral and admitting patients for care to hospitals and aged care.

New roles for nurses and midwives

Many nurses are being employed as on-site staff by mining and other large companies in roles that support the implementation and ongoing management of and compliance with work health and safety policy. In other communities, nurses are accepting positions in primary care settings. General practices are increasingly employing nurses, and there have been added incentives provided by government to support the advancement of practice nurses in these settings (Francis, FitzGerald, Anderson, Mills & Hobbs, 2013). Internationally, nurse practitioners are employed in these settings (Alcolado, 2000; Hoare, Mills & Francis, 2012), and some are practice partners or own the practice. This trend is growing in Australia and will continue to offer nurses other career options.

Advanced practice roles for nurses are occurring in all areas and contexts of practice. Nurses who choose to work in rural areas will continue to be the largest group of health professionals. Changes to healthcare service delivery are likely to impact on nurses' work, with increased utilisation of technologies to diagnose, treat, document and communicate. The provision of healthcare services to isolated and remote communities using telehealth technology coupled with fly-in, fly-out clinics will continue to ensure that all Australians have access to appropriate health care. Nurses have featured – and will continue to feature – in these models of care.

Nurses and midwives will continue to take on clinical leadership roles, and they will need to provide mentorship and clinical supervision to other nurses and midwives to safeguard the future workforce and ensure ongoing sustainability of healthcare services (Mills, Lennon & Francis, 2006). Nurses and midwives must engage with research not only as consumers, but also as contributors to the research agenda and translators of evidence. The public must be confident that the care they access is contemporary and that expected outcomes can be achieved. Being discerning and modifying practice to reflect best practice are advocated and indeed expected. Measuring the impact of nursing and midwifery interventions will continue to be a primary objective of nursing research, particularly rural nursing and midwifery, thus strengthening the evidence that demonstrates the impact of nursing and midwifery care. Nurses and midwives who work in rural contexts will lead change, resulting in the development of appropriate models of care that may result in policy change.

Summary

This chapter provides a summary of the key issues covered in the text. Nurses and midwives who choose to work in rural contexts make a significant contribution to the social and economic fabric of communities. They practise in diverse work settings and are integral to the health and wellbeing of their communities.

Nicole is a new graduate nurse. She grew up in the bush, studied nursing at a regional university and is enthusiastic about working in a rural primary healthcare setting. She has applied for a position in a general practice in a rural town that has a population of 22 000 people. The general practice is a corporate practice that employs two general practitioners (one of whom is an internationally qualified doctor from Uganda), a trainee general practitioner and two practice nurses, one of whom is a registered nurse and the other an enrolled nurse. The practice manager is a woman aged 45 years who has an administration background. The practice has a relationship with a physiotherapist and a podiatrist who offer clinics from the general practice

>> one day a week. The owner has a small hospital, and each of the doctors has visiting medical officer rights to it. Nicole has been told that the practice would like to expand their services to include a clinic for chronic illness management and refugee health. Nicole is particularly interested in chronic and complex care and refugee health.

Nicole wants to undertake an honours degree and has been accepted. Her new employer is supportive of this endeavour and suggests that she looks at her practice to isolate a research project. The general practice manager has confirmed that the practice will provide half a day weekly for her to focus on her study and that they expect she will present a minimum of two seminars to the staff of the practice. Nicole hasn't as yet decided on further career choices, although she is interested in specialising and thinks that she wants to advance her practice and possibly study to become a nurse practitioner.

Questions

1 What preparation should Nicole engage in before commencing work?
2 Discuss the strategies Nicole will need to think about to ensure that her practice meets the general practice's expectations.
3 List methods that Nicole can use to ensure that her practice is contemporary and that she meets the requirements for annual licensing.
4 Working in a multidisciplinary team within a general practice team will be a feature of Nicole's practice. Identify methods that Nicole can utilise to ensure that she is well prepared to work in this environment with such a diverse group of health professionals.
5 Describe ways Nicole could isolate a research topic for her honours degree.
6 What challenges do you think Nicole will encounter as a new graduate nurse?
7 Discuss strategies that Nicole can self-initiate to ensure her success as both a clinician and a researcher.
8 Nicole is keen to advance her practice. What strategies should she consider to achieve this goal?

References

Alcolado, J. (2000). Nurse practitioners and the future of general practice. *British Medical Journal*, 320(1084), 1.

Australian Government. (2012). *National Suicide Prevention Strategy*. Canberra: Australian Government. Retrieved October 31, 2013, from http://www.health. gov.au/internet/main/publishing.nsf/content/mental-nsps

Banks, G. (2005). *Australia's health workforce: Productivity commission research report*. Canberra: Commonwealth of Australia.

beyondblue. (2013). 3 million Australians are living with depression or anxiety. Retrieved October 31, 2013, from http://www.beyondblue.org.au

Francis, K., FitzGerald, M., Anderson, J., Mills, N. & Hobbs, T. (2013). Advanced roles for nurses working in general practice: A study of barriers and enablers for nurses in rural Australia. *Journal of Clinical Nursing Studies*, 1(4), 45–55.

Francis, K. & Mills, J. (2011). Sustaining and growing the rural nursing and midwifery workforce: Understanding the issues and isolating directions for the future. *Collegian*, 18(2), 55–60.

Health Workforce Australia. (2011). *National Health Workforce Innovation and Reform Strategic Framework for Action 2011–2015*. Adelaide: Health Workforce Australia.

——. (2012). *Health Workforce 2025 – Doctors, Nurses and Midwives, Volume 1*. Adelaide: Health Workforce Australia.

Hoare, K. J., Mills, J. & Francis, K. (2012). The role of Government policy in supporting nurse-led care in general practice in the United Kingdom, New Zealand and Australia: An adapted realist review. *Journal of Advanced Nursing*, 68(5), 963–80.

Indigenous Allied Health Australia (IAHA). (2013, October 2). You can lead the way towards being culturally responsive. Paper presented at the *2nd International Allied Health Professionals Conference*, Edinburgh, Scotland.

Keane, B. (2013). The threat of the internet to retail. Retrieved October 25, 2013, from http://www.crikey.com.au/2011/07/27/underestimating-the-threat-of-the-internet-to-retail/

KPMG. (2013). 2013 Retail industry outlook survey. Retrieved October 22, 2013, from http://www.kpmg.com/US/en/IssuesAndInsights/ArticlesPublications/Documents/retail-outlook-survey.pdf

Mills, J., Lennon, D. & Francis, K. (2006). Mentoring matters: Developing rural nurses knowledge and skills. *Collegian*, 13(3), 32–6.

National Rural Health Alliance (NRHA). (2009). Suicide rates in rural Australia. National Rural Health Alliance Fact Sheet 4. Canberra: NRHA.

Nurses and Midwives Accreditation Council. (2012). Australian Nursing and Midwifery Accreditation Council (ANMAC). Retrieved February 27, 2012, from http://www.anmc.org.au

ReachOut. (2013). Suicide. Retrieved October 31, 2013, from http://au.reachout.com/Tough-Times/Physical-health/Suicide?gclid=CPqHxoDbv7oCFQtDpAoddxIAXg

Suicide Prevention Australia. (2013). Communities matter. Retrieved October 31, 2013, from http://suicidepreventionaust.org/about/

Index

Printed in the United States
By Bookmasters